Table of Contents

Table of Content 1
Chapter 1: Introduction 2
Chapter 2: Warming Up and Getting Ready 13
Chapter 3: Building a Strong Core 23
Chapter 4: Sculpting Your Arms 32
Chapter 5: Defining Your Shoulders 40
Chapter 6: Advanced Wall Workouts 48
Chapter 7: Understanding Your Body's Feedback 58
Chapter 8: Adapting Workouts for Different Levels 67
Chapter 9: Incorporating Wall Workouts into Your Routine 75
Chapter 10: Nutrition for Upper Body Strength 83
Chapter 11: Rest and Recovery 91
Chapter 12: Addressing Common Upper Body Concerns 100
Chapter 13: Maximizing Your Results 111
Chapter 14: Beyond the Wall: Exploring Other Pilates Exercises
.... 120
Chapter 15: Maintaining Strength and Sculpting a Defined Physique 130
Chapter 16: Conclusion 139

Chapter 1: Introduction

1.1 The Power of Wall Workouts

Wall workouts, often overlooked in the fitness realm, possess a remarkable array of benefits that cater to individuals of diverse fitness levels and goals. Their versatility allows for customization and progression, making them suitable for both beginners and seasoned fitness enthusiasts.

1.1.1 Accessibility and Space Efficiency

Wall workouts are highly accessible, requiring minimal equipment and space. They can be performed virtually anywhere with a wall, whether at home, in a gym, or even outdoors. This accessibility makes them ideal for individuals with limited time, space, or access to traditional fitness facilities.

1.1.2 Bodyweight Training

Many wall workouts utilize bodyweight as resistance, eliminating the need for weights or machines. Bodyweight training is advantageous as it allows for personalized resistance based on an individual's weight and fitness level. It also promotes functional movements that engage multiple muscle groups simultaneously.

1.1.3 Improved Posture and Balance

Wall workouts often involve exercises that require maintaining a neutral spine and proper alignment against the wall. This helps improve posture, reduce muscular imbalances, and enhance overall stability. Additionally, exercises like wall sits and leg raises challenge balance and coordination, fostering better body control.

1.1.4 Variety and Customization

Wall workouts offer a wide range of exercises that target different muscle groups and movement patterns. This variety allows for comprehensive full-body workouts or focused training sessions for specific areas. The exercises can be modified to adjust difficulty, making them suitable for both beginners and advanced athletes.

1.1.5 Reduced Risk of Injury

Wall workouts can be less strenuous on joints and muscles compared to some traditional weightlifting exercises. The wall provides support and stability, reducing the risk of injuries caused by improper form or excessive weight. This makes them a viable option for individuals with pre-existing injuries or those seeking a lower-impact workout.

Sample Wall Workout:

To experience the benefits of wall workouts, consider incorporating these exercises into your fitness routine:

Wall sit: Stand with your back against the wall, feet hip-width apart and thighs parallel to the floor. Hold for 30-60 seconds.
Wall push-up: Position your hands shoulder-width apart against the wall, step back, and lower your chest towards

the wall. Perform 10-15 repetitions.

Leg raises: Lie on your back with your legs extended towards the wall. Lift one leg towards the wall, keeping your core engaged. Lower and repeat with the other leg. Aim for 10-15 repetitions per leg.

Plank: Place your forearms on the wall, shoulder-width apart, and step back into a plank position. Hold for 30-60 seconds.

Calf raises: Stand facing the wall with your feet flat on the floor. Raise up onto your toes, lifting your heels towards the wall. Lower and repeat for 15-20 repetitions.

Conclusion

Wall workouts are a versatile and effective way to improve fitness, regardless of your experience level. They offer accessibility, bodyweight resistance, posture enhancement, and a wide range of exercises. Whether you're a beginner looking to start your fitness journey or an experienced athlete seeking new challenges, incorporating wall workouts into your routine can help you achieve your fitness goals.

1.2 Benefits of Pilates for Upper Body Strength

Pilates, a mind-body exercise method created by Joseph Pilates in the early 20th century, has gained immense popularity in recent years due to its numerous physical and mental benefits. Initially developed as a rehabilitation program for injured dancers, Pilates has evolved into a comprehensive exercise system that caters to individuals of all ages and fitness levels. This holistic approach focuses on strengthening the core, improving flexibility, and enhancing body awareness.

Benefits of Pilates for Upper Body Strength

Pilates offers a myriad of benefits for upper body strength. Regular practice can help individuals:

1. Strengthen Shoulders and Back:

Pilates exercises effectively target the muscles of the shoulders and back, including the trapezius, rhomboids, and latissimus dorsi. These muscles are crucial for maintaining good posture, preventing shoulder pain, and improving overall upper body mobility.

2. Improve Posture:

Strong upper body muscles contribute to proper posture by aligning the spine and reducing slouching. Pilates exercises specifically designed to strengthen the shoulder girdle and back help individuals develop a strong and balanced posture.

3. Reduce Risk of Injuries:

Strengthening the upper body muscles can help reduce the risk of injuries, particularly those related to sports or repetitive activities. Well-developed shoulder and back muscles provide stability and support, protecting against strains, sprains, and other musculoskeletal issues.

4. Enhance Functional Movement:

Strong upper body muscles are essential for everyday functional movements, such as lifting, reaching, and pushing. Pilates exercises improve the strength and coordination of these muscles, making daily tasks easier and more efficient.

5. Increase Bone Density:

Resistance exercises like Pilates have been shown to increase bone density, which is particularly important for women and individuals at risk of osteoporosis. Strengthening the upper body muscles can help maintain strong and healthy bones.

Specific Pilates Exercises for Upper Body Strength

Numerous Pilates exercises target and strengthen the upper body muscles. Some of the most effective exercises include:

1. Hundred:

This dynamic exercise engages the core and shoulder muscles. Lying on the mat with the legs extended, lift the head and shoulders off the ground while pumping the arms up and down in a controlled motion.

2. Roll-Up:

Starting in a seated position, slowly roll up to a standing position, engaging the abdominal muscles and the erector spinae in the back. This exercise strengthens the entire back and core.

3. Swan Dive:

Lying face down on the mat, lift the chest and legs off the ground simultaneously. This exercise targets the back extensors and shoulder muscles.

4. Side Plank:

Supporting the body on one forearm and the side of the

foot, hold the position with the core engaged and the back in a straight line. This exercise strengthens the lateral muscles of the back and abdomen.

5. Shoulder Bridge:

Lying on the mat with the knees bent and feet flat on the ground, lift the hips off the ground. This exercise targets the glutes and the upper back muscles.

Conclusion

Pilates offers a comprehensive and effective approach to strengthening the upper body. By engaging in regular Pilates practice, individuals can enhance their shoulder and back strength, improve their posture, reduce the risk of injuries, and improve their overall functional movement. The specific exercises mentioned in this article provide a foundation for developing a stronger and more resilient upper body. It is important to note that proper form and technique are crucial to ensure safety and maximize the benefits of Pilates.

1.3 Understanding the Principles of Pilates

Introduction:
Pilates, a mind-body exercise method developed by Joseph Pilates in the early 20th century, has gained widespread popularity for its comprehensive approach to physical fitness and overall well-being. Understanding the core principles of Pilates is crucial for effective practice and maximizing its benefits.

Principles of Pilates:
Joseph Pilates established six fundamental principles that guide the practice of Pilates:

1. Concentration: Maintaining focus and mental engagement throughout the exercises to enhance precision and maximize results.

2. Control: Executing movements with deliberate control and awareness, allowing for targeted muscle engagement and avoiding excessive strain.

3. Centering: Engaging the core muscles (abdominals, lower back, and pelvic floor) to stabilize and support the body during exercises.

4. Flow: Performing movements seamlessly and rhythmically, connecting mind and body for increased coordination and fluidity.

5. Precision: Aiming for accuracy and detail in movement execution, ensuring proper form and minimizing the risk of injury.

6. Breathing: Coordinating breath with movement to oxygenate the body, enhance endurance, and promote relaxation.

Core Concepts:
Beyond the six principles, several core concepts underpin the Pilates method:

1. Neutral Spine: Maintaining a neutral spinal alignment throughout exercises, protecting the spine and reducing stress on the joints.

2. Pelvic Tilt: Tilting the pelvis posteriorly to engage the lower back muscles and reduce lumbar lordosis (excessive inward curvature).

3. Scapular Stabilization: Stabilizing the shoulder blades to prevent excessive mobility and promote proper shoulder function.

4. Longitudinal Stretching: Lengthening the muscles through controlled movements, improving flexibility and range of motion.

5. Isolation: Focusing on specific muscle groups in isolation to enhance strength and stability in targeted areas.

Integration of Principles and Concepts:
The principles and concepts of Pilates work synergistically to guide practitioners towards effective exercise. For example, maintaining concentration and control during pelvic tilts ensures precise engagement of the lower back muscles. Similarly, flowing movements with proper breathing facilitate seamless transitions and enhance endurance.

Benefits of Pilates:
Adhering to the principles of Pilates provides numerous physical and mental benefits:

1. Improved Posture and Alignment: Strengthened core muscles promote proper posture and spinal alignment, reducing pain and improving overall body mechanics.

2. Enhanced Core Strength and Stability: Pilates exercises target and strengthen the core muscles, providing support for the back, pelvis, and hips.

3. Increased Flexibility and Range of Motion: Longitudinal stretching exercises enhance flexibility in the muscles and joints, promoting ease of movement and reducing the risk of injury.

4. Improved Balance and Coordination: Pilates exercises challenge balance and coordination, fostering increased awareness of body position and movement.

5. Stress Reduction and Relaxation: The focus on breathing and controlled movements promotes relaxation and reduces stress levels. By adhering to the principles and core concepts, individuals can effectively target specific muscle groups, improve posture, enhance flexibility, and reduce stress. Pilates provides a comprehensive and adaptable exercise method that caters to diverse fitness levels and can be integrated into any fitness routine.

1.4 Getting Started with Wall Workouts

Wall workouts are an accessible and effective way to improve your fitness, regardless of your age or fitness level. They require minimal equipment and can be done anywhere, making them a convenient option for those with busy schedules or limited access to a gym.

Benefits of Wall Workouts

Wall workouts offer numerous benefits, including:

Improved strength and endurance: Wall exercises engage multiple muscle groups, helping to build strength and endurance in your arms, legs, core, and back.
Enhanced flexibility: Holding various positions against a wall helps to improve flexibility in your muscles and joints.
Reduced risk of injury: Proper form and technique are essential in wall workouts, reducing the risk of injuries.
Increased mobility: Wall exercises can help improve your range of motion and overall mobility.
Convenience and accessibility: Wall workouts can be done anywhere with no special equipment, making them a

convenient and accessible form of exercise.

Getting Started with Wall Workouts

To get started with wall workouts, follow these steps:

1. Choose a suitable wall: Select a sturdy wall with a smooth surface. Avoid using walls with uneven surfaces or sharp edges.
2. Warm up: Before starting your workout, warm up by performing light cardio exercises, such as jumping jacks or high knees, for 5-10 minutes. This will prepare your muscles for the workout.
3. Start gradually: Begin with simple exercises that target your major muscle groups. Gradually increase the intensity and duration of your workouts as you get stronger.
4. Pay attention to form: Proper form is crucial to prevent injuries and maximize the effectiveness of the exercises. Focus on maintaining a neutral spine, engaging your core, and using proper breathing techniques.
5. Rest and recovery: Rest for 60-90 seconds between sets and 2-3 minutes between exercises. This will allow your muscles to recover and prevent overtraining.

Sample Wall Workout

Here is a sample wall workout for beginners:

Wall Push-ups: 10-15 repetitions
Wall Squats: 15-20 repetitions
Wall Sit Hold: 30-60 seconds
Wall Calf Raises: 15-20 repetitions
Wall Plank: 30-60 seconds

Repeat this circuit 2-3 times, resting for 60-90 seconds between sets.

Tips for Wall Workouts

Listen to your body: If you experience any pain or discomfort, stop the exercise and consult with a healthcare professional.
Stay hydrated: Drink plenty of water before, during, and after your workout.
Find a workout buddy: Having a workout partner can provide motivation and accountability.
Have fun: Wall workouts should be enjoyable. Choose exercises that you like and that challenge you.

Conclusion

Wall workouts are a versatile and effective form of exercise that can benefit individuals of all fitness levels. By following proper form, starting gradually, and paying attention to your body, you can reap the numerous benefits of wall workouts, including improved strength, endurance, flexibility, and mobility.

Chapter 2: Warming Up and Getting Ready

2.1 Importance of Warming Up

Before delving into the intricacies of physical activity and exercise, it is imperative to underscore the paramount significance of warming up. Warming up prepares the body for the rigors of exercise, ensuring optimal performance and minimizing the risk of injury. It is an essential component of any exercise routine, regardless of fitness level or the intensity of the activity.

The primary goal of warming up is to elevate the body's core temperature, increasing blood flow to the muscles. This process facilitates the delivery of oxygen and nutrients to the muscles, enhancing their ability to contract efficiently and generate force. Warming up also increases the elasticity of connective tissues, such as tendons and ligaments, reducing the likelihood of strains and tears.

There are two main types of warm-ups: general and specific. General warm-ups involve low-intensity, full-body movements that gradually increase the heart rate and body temperature. Examples of general warm-ups include light jogging, cycling, or jumping jacks. Specific warm-ups, on the other hand, are tailored to the specific activity that will be performed. They involve movements that mimic the actions of the main exercise, gradually increasing the range of motion and intensity. For instance, if the main activity is running, a specific warm-up might include dynamic stretches for the legs and core, as well as practice strides.

The duration and intensity of a warm-up depend on the individual and the activity being performed. As a general rule, a warm-up should last for 5-10 minutes and should be tailored to the individual's fitness level. For low-intensity activities, such as walking or light cycling, a shorter and less intense warm-up may be sufficient. Conversely, for high-intensity activities, such as sprinting or weightlifting, a longer and more intense warm-up is necessary.

There is ample scientific evidence to support the benefits of warming up before exercise. Studies have shown that warming up can:

Improve performance: Warming up has been shown to enhance muscle power, endurance, and coordination. This is particularly important for activities that require explosive movements, such as sprinting or jumping.
Reduce the risk of injury: Warming up helps to prepare the body for the stresses of exercise, reducing the risk of strains, sprains, and other injuries.
Improve recovery: Warming up can help to reduce muscle soreness and stiffness after exercise, facilitating faster recovery.

In addition to these physiological benefits, warming up also has psychological benefits. It can help to focus the mind and prepare the individual mentally for the challenges of exercise. It can also create a sense of routine and consistency, making exercise more enjoyable and sustainable.

In summary, warming up is an indispensable component of any exercise routine. It prepares the body for the rigors of exercise, enhances performance, reduces the risk of injury, improves recovery, and provides psychological benefits. By incorporating a proper warm-up into every workout, individuals can maximize their results and minimize the chances of setbacks.

2.2 Dynamic Stretches for Upper Body

Dynamic stretching involves active movements that mimic the motions used in your specific sport or activity. Unlike static stretching, which holds a position for a prolonged period, dynamic stretching prepares your body for movement by increasing range of motion, improving coordination, and enhancing muscular power.

Benefits of Dynamic Stretches for Upper Body:

1. Increased Range of Motion: Dynamic stretches gently guide your muscles and joints through their full range of motion, gradually increasing their flexibility and allowing for more efficient movement during athletic activities.

2. Improved Coordination: Dynamic stretches involve controlled and purposeful movements that enhance neuromuscular coordination, enabling better communication between your muscles and nervous system. This improved coordination leads to smoother and more efficient movements.

3. Enhanced Muscular Power: By engaging your muscles in dynamic movements, these stretches activate and prime them for explosive actions, improving muscular power and explosiveness, essential for activities like sprinting, jumping, or throwing.

4. Reduced Risk of Injury: Dynamic stretches help prepare

your muscles and connective tissues for the demands of physical activity, reducing the risk of strains, sprains, or other injuries that can arise from sudden or forceful movements.

Effective Dynamic Stretches for Upper Body:

1. Arm Circles: Stand with your feet shoulder-width apart and your arms extended to the sides at shoulder height. Rotate your arms in small circles, gradually increasing the diameter of the circles. Continue for 30-60 seconds.

2. Shoulder Rolls: Stand or sit upright and roll your shoulders forward in a circular motion for 30-60 seconds. Reverse the direction and roll your shoulders backward for another 30-60 seconds.

3. Arm Swings: Stand with your feet shoulder-width apart and your arms relaxed at your sides. Swing your arms forward and backward, increasing the range of motion gradually. Continue for 30-60 seconds.

4. Wall Slides: Stand facing a wall with your feet hip-width apart and your hands placed on the wall at shoulder height. Step away from the wall until your arms are fully extended. Slide your body down the wall until your chest touches the wall. Hold for a few seconds and then push yourself back up to the starting position. Repeat for 10-15 repetitions.

5. Elbow Extensions: Stand or sit with your feet flat on the floor and your elbows bent at 90 degrees, palms facing up. Extend your arms overhead, keeping your elbows slightly bent. Return to the starting position and repeat for 10-15 repetitions.

6. Triceps Extensions: Stand or sit with your feet flat on the

floor and your elbows bent at 90 degrees, palms facing your body. Extend your elbows backward, keeping your upper arms stationary. Return to the starting position and repeat for 10-15 repetitions.

7. Wrist Flexions and Extensions: Stand or sit with your feet flat on the floor and your arms extended in front of you. Flex your wrists forward and hold for a few seconds. Then, extend your wrists backward and hold for a few seconds. Repeat for 10-15 repetitions.

8. Rotator Cuff Stretches: Stand or sit with your feet flat on the floor and your arms extended to the sides at shoulder height. Rotate your arms inward, crossing them in front of your chest. Hold for a few seconds and then rotate your arms outward, extending them behind you. Repeat for 10-15 repetitions.

Incorporating Dynamic Stretches into Your Routine:

Dynamic stretches should be performed as part of your warm-up routine before engaging in physical activity. Start with gentle movements and gradually increase the intensity and range of motion as your body warms up. Aim for 5-10 minutes of dynamic stretching before your workout or sport.

2.3 Choosing the Right Wall Space

Selecting the ideal wall space for your artwork is a crucial step in showcasing your collection effectively. The size, shape, and location of the wall space will influence the overall impact of the artwork and how it interacts with the surrounding environment. Here are some key considerations to guide your decision-making process:

1. Size and Shape of the Wall Space:

The size and shape of the wall space will determine the scale and orientation of the artwork you choose. A large, expansive wall can accommodate a series of smaller pieces or a single, monumental work. Conversely, a smaller wall space may require a more compact or vertical arrangement. Consider the proportions of the wall and the relationship between the artwork's height and width.

2. Natural and Artificial Lighting:

The quality and direction of lighting can dramatically affect the appearance of artwork. Natural light provides a warm, diffused glow, while artificial light can create more dramatic effects. Assess the natural light sources in the room, such as windows or skylights, and determine how they will interact with the artwork. Consider the time of day and the potential for glare or shadows.

3. Background Color and Texture:

The color and texture of the wall behind the artwork can significantly influence its visual impact. A neutral-colored wall, such as white or gray, can provide a clean and unobtrusive backdrop, allowing the artwork to take center stage. Conversely, a patterned or textured wall can create a more dynamic and engaging context for the pieces.

4. Surrounding Environment:

The surounding environment, including furniture, décor, and architectural features, can influence the perception of the artwork. Consider how the artwork will interact with nearby objects and whether it will complement or contrast with the existing design scheme. Ensure that there is sufficient space around the artwork to allow viewers to appreciate it without distractions.

5. Viewing Distance:

The viewing distance, or the distance from which the artwork will be observed, should be taken into account when selecting wall space. Larger artworks require a greater viewing distance, while smaller pieces can be viewed from a closer range. Determine the ideal viewing distance for the artwork and choose a wall space that allows viewers to engage with it comfortably.

6. Focal Point:

If you have multiple artworks to display, consider creating a focal point within the composition. The focal point should be the most prominent or eye-catching piece, and it should be placed in a central or prominent location on the wall. Arrange the remaining artworks around the focal point to create a cohesive and balanced display.

7. Grouping and Arrangement:

The grouping and arrangement of the artwork on the wall can enhance its visual impact. Experiment with different arrangements, considering the size, shape, and colors of the pieces. Create groupings based on common themes, styles, or periods. Use spacing and alignment to create a dynamic and visually pleasing composition.

8. Personal Preference:

Ultimately, the choice of wall space should reflect your personal taste and preferences. Consider the intended mood and atmosphere you want to create with the artwork. Experiment with different arrangements and lighting conditions until you find a solution that resonates with your sensibilities.

2.4 Essential Equipment: Mat, Pillow, and Resistance Bands

The Pilates Mat: A Foundation for Body Awareness

The Pilates mat is the cornerstone of any Pilates practice. It provides a stable and supportive surface that allows practitioners to focus on their body movements and alignment without the added challenges of balance. The mat's firm yet yielding texture encourages proper spinal alignment, promotes stability, and cushions joints during exercises. Its portability makes it an ideal companion for home workouts or travel.

Benefits of the Pilates Mat:

Enhances body awareness by providing a stable surface
Promotes proper spinal alignment and postural correction
Cushions joints and reduces strain
Encourages precision and control in movements
Ideal for home workouts and travel

Choosing the Right Pilates Mat:

Thickness: Choose a mat that is thick enough (6mm or more) to provide sufficient cushioning without being too soft.
Texture: Opt for a mat with a non-slip texture to prevent sliding during workouts.
Size: Select a mat that is large enough to accommodate your body comfortably.
Material: Choose a mat made from durable and non-toxic materials for longevity and safety.

The Pilates Pillow: Support for Lumbar and Spine

The Pilates pillow is a versatile tool that provides support and alignment in various Pilates exercises. It can be placed under the head, neck, or back to promote proper spinal curvature, reduce strain, and enhance comfort. The pillow's soft yet firm texture allows for gentle support without compromising movement range.

Benefits of the Pilates Pillow:

Supports the head, neck, and back
Maintains proper spinal curvature
Reduces strain and discomfort
Enhances comfort during exercises
Ideal for both beginners and experienced practitioners

Choosing the Right Pilates Pillow:

Shape: Choose a pillow that is designed specifically for Pilates, with a contoured shape to provide optimal support.
Firmness: Opt for a pillow that is firm enough to provide support without being too rigid.
Size: Select a pillow that is proportional to your body size and the exercises you plan to do.
Material: Choose a pillow made from durable and comfortable materials that won't flatten or lose shape over time.

Resistance Bands: Enhance Strength and Flexibility

Resistance bands are elastic bands that provide variable resistance during exercises. They can be used to enhance strength, improve flexibility, and support rehabilitation. By adjusting the tension of the band, practitioners can tailor the difficulty to suit their individual fitness levels.

Resistance bands are lightweight, portable, and affordable, making them a versatile addition to any fitness routine.

Benefits of Resistance Bands:

Enhance muscular strength and endurance
Improve flexibility and range of motion
Support rehabilitation and injury prevention
Can be used for a wide range of exercises
Compact and easy to transport

Choosing the Right Resistance Bands:

Resistance Level: Choose bands with resistance levels that challenge you without compromising form.
Material: Opt for bands made from durable and non-toxic materials to ensure longevity and safety.
Size: Select bands that are long enough to accommodate various exercises and body sizes.
Attachment Points: Choose bands with sturdy attachment points to prevent breakage or slippage.

Chapter 3: Building a Strong Core

3.1 The Core as the Foundation of Upper Body Strength

The core, often referred to as the powerhouse of the body, serves as the central link between the upper and lower body. It comprises an intricate network of muscles, including the abdominal muscles (rectus abdominis, external/internal obliques, transverse abdominis), back muscles (erector spinae, latissimus dorsi), and pelvic floor muscles. These muscles work synergistically to stabilize the spine, pelvis, and rib cage, creating a solid foundation for efficient movement patterns.

In the context of upper body strength, a strong core plays a pivotal role in generating power and maintaining stability during various exercises. Here's how the core contributes to upper body strength:

1. Stabilization and Control:

A strong core acts as a stabilizing force for the upper body, preventing excessive movement and maintaining proper alignment during exercises. For instance, during a bench press, the core muscles engage to stabilize the spine, preventing it from arching excessively, which could lead to injury or reduced force production. Similarly, in overhead presses, the core provides stability to the shoulder girdle, enabling optimal positioning and force generation.

2. Force Transfer:

The core muscles facilitate force transfer between the lower and upper body. During exercises like squats and deadlifts, the core contracts to transfer force from the lower body to the upper body, aiding in the lifting motion. Conversely, in exercises like pull-ups or rows, the core helps transmit force from the upper body to the lower body, facilitating the pulling action.

3. Power Generation:

A strong core is essential for generating explosive power in upper body exercises. During exercises like plyometric push-ups or medicine ball slams, the core muscles engage to generate force and contribute to the rapid and forceful movements required for these exercises. The core muscles act as a springboard, absorbing and releasing energy to enhance power output.

4. Improved Breathing Mechanics:

The core muscles, particularly the diaphragm and transverse abdominis, play a crucial role in breathing. During heavy upper body exercises, maintaining proper breathing is essential for oxygen delivery and waste product removal. A strong core ensures efficient breathing mechanics, allowing for optimal gas exchange and reducing fatigue.

5. Injury Prevention:

A strong core helps prevent injuries by providing stability and support to the spine and pelvis. By maintaining proper alignment and reducing excessive movement, the core muscles protect the spine from strain, herniated discs, and other injuries. Additionally, a strong core can enhance balance and coordination, reducing the risk of falls and accidents during upper body exercises.

Training the Core for Upper Body Strength:

To develop a strong core that supports upper body strength, it's crucial to incorporate regular core training into your fitness routine. Here are some effective exercises to target the core muscles:

Planks: Hold a position with your forearms and toes on the ground, keeping your body in a straight line from head to heels. Engage your core to stabilize your body and hold for 30-60 seconds.
Crunches: Lie on your back with knees bent and feet flat on the floor. Contract your abdominal muscles to lift your head and shoulders off the ground, then slowly lower back down.
Leg Raises: Lie on your back with your legs extended straight up. Keep your lower back pressed into the ground and slowly lower your legs until they are parallel to the ground, then raise them back up.
Bird Dogs: Start on your hands and knees. Extend your right arm forward and your left leg backward simultaneously, keeping your core engaged and your back flat. Hold for a few seconds, then return to the starting position and repeat with the opposite arm and leg.
Russian Twists: Sit on the floor with your knees bent and feet elevated slightly. Hold a weight in front of your chest and twist your torso from side to side, engaging your obliques.

Remember to start with a manageable level of intensity and gradually increase the difficulty as you progress. Proper form is essential to prevent injuries and maximize the effectiveness of the exercises. Consult with a qualified fitness professional for guidance on proper technique and personalized training recommendations.

3.2 Pilates Exercises for Core Engagement

Pilates is a low-impact exercise method that emphasizes core engagement, flexibility, and strength. It was developed by Joseph Pilates in the early 20th century as a way to rehabilitate injured soldiers. Pilates exercises are typically performed on a mat or with specialized equipment, such as the Reformer, Cadillac, and Wunda Chair.

The core muscles are the muscles of the abdomen, lower back, and pelvis. They are responsible for stabilizing the spine, pelvis, and shoulder girdle, and for generating movement. Strong core muscles are essential for good posture, balance, and coordination. They also help to protect the spine from injury.

Pilates exercises are designed to target the core muscles in a variety of ways. Some exercises, such as the Hundred, focus on isolating the core muscles and contracting them against resistance. Other exercises, such as the Roll-Up, work the core muscles in a more dynamic way, while also challenging the flexibility and strength of the spine.

Pilates exercises can be modified to suit people of all fitness levels. Beginners should start with basic exercises, such as the Hundred and the Roll-Up, and gradually progress to more challenging exercises as they get stronger. It is important to listen to your body and stop if you experience any pain.

Pilates is a safe and effective way to improve core strength, flexibility, and posture. It is a great exercise method for people of all ages and fitness levels.

Here are some of the benefits of Pilates exercises for core engagement:

Improved posture
Reduced back pain
Increased flexibility
Enhanced balance and coordination
Stronger core muscles
Reduced risk of injury

If you are new to Pilates, it is important to find a qualified instructor who can teach you the proper form and technique. Pilates exercises should be performed with precision and control to be effective.

Here are some tips for getting started with Pilates:

Start with basic exercises and gradually progress to more challenging exercises as you get stronger.
Focus on isolating the core muscles and contracting them against resistance.
Keep your movements slow and controlled.
Breathe deeply throughout the exercises.
Stop if you experience any pain.

Pilates is a great way to improve your core strength, flexibility, and posture. It is a safe and effective exercise method for people of all ages and fitness levels.

3.3 Developing Stability and Control

In the realm of aircraft design, stability and control are paramount considerations that ensure the safe and predictable operation of an aircraft. Stability refers to an aircraft's ability to return to equilibrium after being disturbed, while control denotes the pilot's capability to maneuver the aircraft as desired. Developing and maintaining stability and control are crucial aspects of aircraft design, requiring a comprehensive understanding of aerodynamic principles and careful attention to the aircraft's configuration.

3.3.1 Longitudinal Stability and Control

Longitudinal stability and control concern the aircraft's behavior in the pitch axis, primarily involving the motion of the aircraft's nose up or down. The key parameter in longitudinal stability is the static margin, which is a measure of the aircraft's tendency to return to its equilibrium pitch attitude after a disturbance. A positive static margin indicates that the aircraft will return to its equilibrium, while a negative static margin implies instability.

Maintaining longitudinal stability is essential for preventing the aircraft from entering a dangerous nose-down or nose-up attitude. To achieve this, designers carefully balance the aircraft's center of gravity (CG) relative to the aerodynamic center (AC). The CG is the point at which the aircraft's weight acts, while the AC is the point at which the aerodynamic forces act. A stable aircraft has its CG located behind the AC, ensuring that any disturbance will cause the aircraft to pitch nose-up, bringing it back to its equilibrium.

In addition to static stability, longitudinal control is crucial for maneuvering the aircraft. The primary control surface for longitudinal control is the elevator, located at the tail of the aircraft. Moving the elevator up or down changes the aircraft's angle of attack, causing it to pitch up or down accordingly. Proper design of the elevator ensures that the pilot has adequate control over the aircraft's pitch attitude.

3.3.2 Lateral Stability and Control

Lateral stability and control involve the aircraft's behavior in the roll and yaw axes, primarily concerning the motion of the aircraft's wings and tail. Lateral stability ensures that the aircraft will return to its wings-level attitude after being disturbed, while lateral control allows the pilot to maneuver the aircraft in roll and yaw.

Lateral stability is primarily maintained through the dihedral effect, which is the tendency of an aircraft's wings to tilt downward when the aircraft rolls. This effect creates a restoring moment that brings the aircraft back to its wings-level attitude. The dihedral angle, which is the angle between the wing and the horizontal, determines the strength of the dihedral effect. A larger dihedral angle results in greater lateral stability.

Lateral control is achieved through a combination of ailerons and rudder. Ailerons, located on the trailing edge of the wings, move differentially to create a rolling moment, causing the aircraft to roll left or right. The rudder, located at the tail, controls the aircraft's yaw motion. Moving the rudder left or right creates a yawing moment, causing the aircraft to turn in the desired direction.

3.3.3 Control Surfaces and Systems

Control surfaces are movable aerodynamic surfaces that enable the pilot to maneuver the aircraft. The primary control surfaces are the elevators, ailerons, and rudder, which control the aircraft's pitch, roll, and yaw, respectively. These surfaces are actuated by control systems, which transmit the pilot's inputs to the control surfaces.

Control systems can be mechanical, hydraulic, or electrical. Mechanical control systems use cables or pushrods to connect the control yoke or pedals to the control surfaces. Hydraulic control systems use hydraulic fluid to transmit force from the pilot's controls to the control surfaces. Electrical control systems use electrical signals to actuate the control surfaces.

Modern aircraft typically employ fly-by-wire (FBW) control systems, where electrical signals are used to control the aircraft's flight control surfaces. FBW systems offer numerous advantages, including increased precision, reliability, and redundancy. They also allow for the implementation of advanced flight control laws that improve the aircraft's stability and handling qualities.

3.3.4 Flight Control Laws

Flight control laws are algorithms that govern the behavior of an aircraft's control surfaces. These laws determine how the control surfaces respond to pilot inputs and aircraft states. Flight control laws can be designed to enhance stability, improve handling qualities, or perform specific maneuvers.

Modern aircraft often employ sophisticated flight control laws that incorporate feedback from various sensors to adjust the control surface deflections in real-time. This enables the aircraft to maintain stability and control even in challenging flight conditions, such as high winds or turbulence.

Conclusion

Developing stability and control is a critical aspect of aircraft design, ensuring the safe and predictable operation of the aircraft. By understanding the principles of longitudinal and lateral stability and control, designers can configure aircraft with the appropriate aerodynamic characteristics and control systems. Flight control laws further enhance stability and handling qualities, enabling aircraft to perform complex maneuvers and operate in a wide range of flight conditions.

Chapter 4: Sculpting Your Arms

4.1 Wall Workouts for Triceps and Biceps

Wall workouts are a versatile and effective way to work out your triceps and biceps, two important muscle groups for everyday activities and athletic performance. Here's a detailed guide to help you get started:

Tricep Dips

Stand facing a sturdy wall, with your feet shoulder-width apart and your hands placed on the wall slightly wider than your shoulders.
Step back until your body is in a slight incline.
Bend your elbows to lower your chest towards the wall, keeping your back straight and your core engaged.
Push back up to the starting position using your triceps.
Aim for 10-15 repetitions for 3 sets.

Incline Tricep Push-Ups

Place your hands on the wall slightly higher than shoulder-width apart, with your feet on the floor.
Walk your feet back until your body is in a diagonal line.
Lower your chest towards the wall by bending your elbows, keeping your back straight.
Push back up to the starting position using your triceps.
Aim for 10-15 repetitions for 3 sets.

Bicep Curls

Stand facing the wall, with your feet shoulder-width apart and your hands on the wall slightly lower than shoulder-width apart.
Bend your elbows to curl your hands towards your shoulders, keeping your upper arms stationary.
Slowly lower your hands back to the starting position.
Aim for 10-15 repetitions for 3 sets.

Hammer Curls

Stand facing the wall, with your feet shoulder-width apart and your hands on the wall slightly wider than shoulder-width apart.
Bend your elbows to curl your hands towards your shoulders, keeping your forearms perpendicular to the wall.
Slowly lower your hands back to the starting position.
Aim for 10-15 repetitions for 3 sets.

Wall Sit with Bicep Curls

Stand with your back against the wall, your feet shoulder-width apart, and your hands on the wall slightly wider than shoulder-width apart.
Slowly slide down the wall until your thighs are parallel to the floor.
Hold this position for 30-60 seconds while performing bicep curls.
Aim for 10-15 repetitions for 3 sets.

Benefits of Wall Workouts for Triceps and Biceps

Accessibility: Wall workouts require minimal equipment and can be done anywhere with a sturdy wall.
Versatile: Wall exercises allow for various angles and intensities, accommodating different fitness levels.

Effective: Wall workouts provide a challenging and efficient workout for both the triceps and biceps.
Bodyweight Resistance: Using your own bodyweight as resistance helps develop functional strength and endurance.
Low Impact: Wall exercises are low-impact, making them suitable for individuals with joint issues or injuries.

Tips for Wall Workouts

Use proper form to maximize results and prevent injuries.
Engage your core throughout the exercises to stabilize your body.
Gradually increase the intensity by holding the positions longer or performing more repetitions.
Listen to your body and rest when needed.
Combine wall exercises with other bodyweight exercises for a well-rounded workout.

Conclusion

Incorporating wall workouts into your routine is an excellent way to strengthen and tone your triceps and biceps. Whether you're a beginner or an experienced fitness enthusiast, these exercises offer a versatile and effective way to improve your upper body strength and endurance. Remember to prioritize proper form, listen to your body, and enjoy the process.

4.2 Targeting Specific Muscle Groups

To effectively target specific muscle groups, it's essential to have a foundational understanding of muscle anatomy and physiology. Muscles are composed of bundles of muscle fibers, which contract and relax to generate movement. Each muscle group has a unique origin and insertion point on the skeleton, and its function is determined by the direction of its pull.

For instance, the biceps brachii muscle originates at the scapula (shoulder blade) and inserts at the radius (forearm bone). Its primary function is to flex the elbow joint, bringing the forearm towards the upper arm. Conversely, the triceps brachii muscle originates at the humerus (upper arm bone) and inserts at the ulna (forearm bone). Its primary function is to extend the elbow joint, straightening the forearm.

Targeting Specific Muscle Groups: Isolation and Compound Exercises

When designing a workout program to target specific muscle groups, it's crucial to choose exercises that isolate or compound the desired muscles.

Isolation exercises involve a single joint movement, focusing primarily on one muscle group. For example, the bicep curl isolates the biceps brachii muscle by flexing the elbow joint. Other examples of isolation exercises include the leg extension (isolates the quadriceps) and the calf raise (isolates the gastrocnemius).

Compound exercises, on the other hand, involve multiple joint movements, engaging several muscle groups simultaneously. For example, the squat is a compound exercise that targets the quadriceps, hamstrings, glutes, and calves. Other examples of compound exercises include the bench press (targets the chest, triceps, and shoulders) and the deadlift (targets the hamstrings, glutes, and back).

Exercise Selection and Progression

Selecting the appropriate exercises for targeting specific muscle groups depends on various factors, such as the individual's fitness level, goals, and available equipment. It's advisable to consult with a qualified fitness professional to determine the most suitable exercises and ensure proper form.

Exercise progression is also crucial for continuous improvement. As muscles adapt to a particular resistance, gradually increasing the weight, sets, or repetitions challenges the muscles and stimulates further growth. However, it's essential to progress gradually to avoid overtraining and injuries.

Rest and Recovery

Adequate rest and recovery are vital components of muscle growth and repair. After a workout, muscles require time to rest and rebuild. Sufficient sleep, hydration, and a balanced diet support muscle recovery and prepare the body for subsequent training sessions.

Conclusion

Targeting specific muscle groups requires an understanding of muscle anatomy and physiology, as well as the appropriate selection and progression of exercises. By incorporating isolation and compound exercises into a workout program, individuals can effectively engage and develop specific muscle groups. However, it's crucial to prioritize rest and recovery to facilitate muscle growth and prevent injuries. Consulting with a qualified fitness professional can provide personalized guidance and ensure optimal results.

4.3 Incorporating Resistance Bands for Increased Intensity

Resistance bands, also known as fitness bands or exercise bands, are a versatile and portable piece of fitness equipment that can be used to enhance the intensity of a wide range of exercises. They provide variable resistance, meaning the resistance increases as the band is stretched, making them suitable for users of all fitness levels.

Benefits of Using Resistance Bands

Incorporating resistance bands into your workout routine offers numerous benefits:

Increased muscle activation: Resistance bands create a constant tension on the muscles, leading to greater muscle activation and engagement.
Improved strength and power: The progressive resistance provided by bands challenges the muscles and promotes strength and power development.
Enhanced flexibility: Resistance bands can be used for dynamic stretching exercises, improving flexibility and range of motion.
Reduced risk of injury: Bands provide a gentler form of resistance compared to weights, minimizing the risk of strain or injury.
Versatility: Resistance bands come in various lengths, thicknesses, and resistance levels, allowing for a wide range of exercises and adjustments.
Portability: Bands are lightweight and easy to carry, making them convenient for home workouts or travel.

How to Use Resistance Bands

To effectively incorporate resistance bands into your workouts, follow these guidelines:

Choose the right resistance: Start with a band that provides a challenging but manageable resistance level.
Secure the band: Anchor the band securely to a stable object, such as a doorknob, chair, or workout bench.
Maintain proper form: Focus on maintaining good technique and posture throughout the exercises.
Grasp the band correctly: Hold the handles or ends of the band with a secure grip.
Control the movement: Perform the exercises smoothly and with controlled movements, avoiding sudden jerks or bouncing.

Exercises Using Resistance Bands

Resistance bands can be used for a variety of exercises, targeting different muscle groups. Here are some examples:

Bicep curls: Stand with the band anchored at foot level, grasp the handles with an underhand grip, and curl the band up towards your shoulders.
Tricep extensions: Secure the band overhead, hold the handles with an overhand grip, and extend your arms behind your head.
Lateral raises: Stand on the band with your feet shoulder-width apart, hold the handles by your sides, and raise your arms laterally.
Squats: Place the band around your thighs just above your knees, stand with your feet shoulder-width apart, and perform a squat by lowering your hips towards the ground.
Push-ups: Position the band around your back, hold the handles on the ground, and perform push-ups as usual.

Tips for Beginners

If you're new to using resistance bands, consider these

tips:

Start gradually: Begin with a low resistance band and gradually increase the resistance as you get stronger.
Listen to your body: Rest when necessary and don't push yourself too hard.
Focus on technique: Prioritize proper form over weight or resistance.
Be patient: Building strength and improving fitness takes time and consistency.

Safety Precautions

To ensure a safe and effective workout with resistance bands, follow these precautions:

Inspect the bands regularly for signs of wear or damage.
Avoid overstretching the bands beyond their recommended capacity.
Use the bands on a stable surface to prevent slips or falls.
Consult a healthcare professional if you have any underlying health conditions.

Conclusion

Incorporating resistance bands into your workouts is an effective way to increase intensity, enhance muscle activation, and improve overall fitness. By understanding the benefits, using the bands correctly, and following safety precautions, you can harness the power of resistance bands to achieve your fitness goals safely and effectively.

Chapter 5: Defining Your Shoulders

5.1 Wall Exercises for Shoulder Stability and Mobility

The shoulder is a complex joint that allows for a wide range of motion. However, this mobility also makes it susceptible to instability and injury. Wall exercises can be a safe and effective way to improve shoulder stability and mobility.

Shoulder Stability

Shoulder stability is the ability of the shoulder joint to resist displacement. It is important for preventing shoulder injuries and maintaining optimal function. Wall exercises can help to improve shoulder stability by strengthening the muscles that support the joint.

One of the most important muscles for shoulder stability is the rotator cuff. The rotator cuff is a group of four muscles that surround the shoulder joint. It helps to rotate and stabilize the shoulder, and it also prevents the humerus (upper arm bone) from dislocating.

Wall exercises can help to strengthen the rotator cuff muscles by providing resistance against which the muscles can work. For example, the following exercise can be used to strengthen the external rotator muscles of the shoulder:

Stand facing a wall with your feet shoulder-width apart.

Place your hands on the wall at shoulder height, with your elbows bent at 90 degrees.
Rotate your hands outward against the wall, as if you were trying to turn a doorknob.
Hold the position for 10-15 seconds, then relax.
Repeat 10-15 times.

This exercise can be modified to make it more or less challenging. For example, you can increase the resistance by placing your hands higher on the wall, or you can decrease the resistance by placing your hands lower on the wall.

Shoulder Mobility

Shoulder mobility is the ability of the shoulder joint to move through its full range of motion. It is important for everyday activities such as reaching overhead and throwing. Wall exercises can help to improve shoulder mobility by stretching the muscles that surround the joint.

One of the most important muscles for shoulder mobility is the pectoralis major. The pectoralis major is a large muscle that covers the chest. It helps to flex and adduct the arm, and it also helps to stabilize the shoulder joint.

Wall exercises can help to stretch the pectoralis major muscle by providing resistance against which the muscle can work. For example, the following exercise can be used to stretch the pectoralis major muscle:

Stand facing a wall with your feet shoulder-width apart.
Place your hands on the wall at chest height, with your elbows bent at 90 degrees.
Step forward with your right foot, and lean your body into the wall.
Hold the position for 10-15 seconds, then relax.

Repeat 10-15 times with each leg.

This exercise can be modified to make it more or less challenging. For example, you can increase the stretch by placing your hands higher on the wall, or you can decrease the stretch by placing your hands lower on the wall.

Conclusion

Wall exercises are a safe and effective way to improve shoulder stability and mobility. They can be done at home with minimal equipment, and they can be tailored to individual needs. If you are experiencing shoulder pain or instability, talk to your doctor or physical therapist about whether wall exercises may be right for you.

5.2 Strengthening the Rotator Cuff

The rotator cuff is a group of four muscles that surround the shoulder joint and help to stabilize and rotate the arm. These muscles are the supraspinatus, infraspinatus, teres minor, and subscapularis. The rotator cuff muscles are commonly injured in athletes, especially those who participate in overhead sports such as baseball, tennis, and volleyball.

Rotator cuff injuries can range from mild strains to complete tears. Symptoms of a rotator cuff injury can include pain, stiffness, weakness, and decreased range of motion in the shoulder.

Treatment for a rotator cuff injury typically involves rest, ice, and physical therapy. Physical therapy exercises can help to strengthen the rotator cuff muscles and improve range of motion in the shoulder.

There are a number of exercises that can be used to strengthen the rotator cuff muscles. Some of the most common exercises include:

External rotation: This exercise helps to strengthen the infraspinatus and teres minor muscles. To perform this exercise, sit or stand with your arm at your side and your elbow bent at 90 degrees. Hold a dumbbell or resistance band in your hand and rotate your arm outward, keeping your elbow bent.
Internal rotation: This exercise helps to strengthen the subscapularis muscle. To perform this exercise, sit or stand with your arm at your side and your elbow bent at 90 degrees. Hold a dumbbell or resistance band in your hand and rotate your arm inward, keeping your elbow bent.
Abduction: This exercise helps to strengthen the supraspinatus muscle. To perform this exercise, lie on your side with your arm at your side and your elbow bent at 90 degrees. Hold a dumbbell or resistance band in your hand and lift your arm up and out to the side, keeping your elbow bent.
Flexion: This exercise helps to strengthen all of the rotator cuff muscles. To perform this exercise, sit or stand with your arm at your side and your elbow bent at 90 degrees. Hold a dumbbell or resistance band in your hand and lift your arm up in front of you, keeping your elbow bent.

It is important to start with a light weight or resistance when performing these exercises and to gradually increase the weight or resistance as you get stronger. It is also important to perform these exercises slowly and with control. If you experience any pain while performing these exercises, stop and consult with a doctor or physical therapist.

Strengthening the rotator cuff muscles can help to prevent injuries and improve shoulder function. By following these exercises, you can help to keep your shoulders healthy and strong.

Here are some additional tips for strengthening the rotator cuff:

Warm up before you exercise: Warming up the muscles around your shoulder will help to prevent injuries. Some good warm-up exercises include arm circles, shoulder shrugs, and light cardio.
Cool down after you exercise: Cooling down the muscles around your shoulder will help to reduce soreness and stiffness. Some good cool-down exercises include stretching and light cardio.
Listen to your body: If you experience any pain while performing these exercises, stop and consult with a doctor or physical therapist.
Be patient: Strengthening the rotator cuff muscles takes time and effort. Don't get discouraged if you don't see results immediately. Just keep at it and you will eventually see improvements.

By following these tips, you can help to strengthen your rotator cuff muscles and improve your shoulder function.

5.3 Improving Posture and Reducing Shoulder Pain

Posture refers to the alignment of the body's musculoskeletal system while standing, sitting, or lying down. Maintaining good posture is essential for overall physical health, as it promotes optimal functioning of the musculoskeletal system and prevents strain or injury. Poor posture, on the other hand, can lead to a variety of musculoskeletal problems, including shoulder pain.

The Importance of Maintaining Good Posture

Good posture ensures that the body's weight is distributed evenly across the joints and muscles, reducing the risk of strain or injury. It also helps to maintain proper spinal alignment, which is crucial for optimal nerve and blood flow throughout the body. Additionally, good posture can improve balance, coordination, and flexibility, contributing to overall physical fitness and well-being.

How Poor Posture Contributes to Shoulder Pain

Poor posture can put excessive strain on the muscles, tendons, and ligaments of the shoulder, leading to pain and discomfort. When the shoulders are not properly aligned, the muscles around the shoulder joint have to work harder to maintain stability, resulting in muscle fatigue and strain. This strain can manifest as pain in the shoulder, neck, or upper back.

Improving Posture to Reduce Shoulder Pain

Improving posture is a gradual process that requires conscious effort and consistency. Here are some tips for improving posture and reducing shoulder pain:

1. Be Aware of Your Posture:

Pay attention to your posture throughout the day, particularly when sitting, standing, or walking. Notice if you tend to slouch, hunch your shoulders, or lean forward.

2. Practice Proper Sitting Posture:

When sitting, ensure that your feet are flat on the floor, your knees are bent at a 90-degree angle, and your back is straight. Use a lumbar support pillow to maintain the natural curve of your lower back.

3. Stand Up Straight:

When standing, keep your head held high, your shoulders relaxed, and your spine straight. Avoid locking your knees or leaning to one side. Distribute your weight evenly on both feet.

4. Sleep in a Neutral Position:

When sleeping, lie on your back or side with a pillow under your head and between your knees to support the natural curves of your spine. Avoid sleeping on your stomach, as this can put strain on your neck and shoulders.

5. Strengthen Your Core Muscles:

Strengthening your core muscles, including the abdominal and back muscles, helps to support the spine and maintain good posture. Engage in core-strengthening exercises such as planks, crunches, and bridges.

6. Stretch Regularly:

Regular stretching helps to improve flexibility and reduce muscle tension. Incorporate shoulder stretches into your daily routine, such as arm circles, shoulder rolls, and chest stretches.

7. Use Ergonomic Tools:

When working or engaging in activities that require prolonged sitting or standing, use ergonomic tools such as an adjustable chair, a footrest, and a standing desk to promote good posture.

8. Seek Professional Help if Needed:

If you experience persistent shoulder pain that does not improve with self-care measures, consider consulting a healthcare professional such as a physical therapist or chiropractor. They can assess your posture, identify any underlying musculoskeletal issues, and develop a personalized treatment plan to address the pain.

Conclusion

Maintaining good posture is essential for preventing shoulder pain and promoting overall physical well-being. By being aware of your posture, practicing proper alignment, strengthening your core muscles, stretching regularly, and using ergonomic tools, you can improve your posture and reduce shoulder pain. Remember that improving posture is a gradual process that requires consistency and effort, but the benefits are well worth it.

Chapter 6: Advanced Wall Workouts

6.1 Combining Elements for Comprehensive Upper Body Strengthening

The upper body encompasses a diverse array of muscle groups that work in intricate harmony to execute a myriad of functional movements, ranging from basic daily activities to athletic endeavors. To achieve optimal upper body strength and development, a comprehensive approach that incorporates a variety of exercises targeting different muscle groups is essential. This section delves into the principles of combining exercises for a well-rounded upper body strengthening program.

Synergistic Muscle Group Combinations

Effective upper body strengthening entails targeting multiple muscle groups simultaneously through compound exercises. These exercises allow for greater efficiency and time optimization. By combining synergistic muscle groups, such as the chest and triceps or the back and biceps, you can stimulate multiple muscles with a single movement.

For instance, the barbell bench press is a compound exercise that primarily targets the chest (pectoralis major and minor). However, it also engages the triceps and anterior deltoids (front shoulders) as secondary movers. This synergistic action allows for comprehensive upper body development with a single exercise.

Isolation Exercises for Targeted Development

While compound exercises form the foundation of an upper body strengthening program, isolation exercises play a crucial role in targeting specific muscle groups. Isolation exercises focus on a single muscle or muscle group, allowing for isolated development and refinement.

An example of an isolation exercise is the bicep curl. This exercise primarily targets the biceps brachii, the muscle responsible for flexing the elbow. By isolating this muscle group, you can emphasize its development and improve its strength and definition.

Progressive Overload and Variation

To continually challenge your muscles and promote continuous growth, it is imperative to implement progressive overload. This principle involves gradually increasing the weight, resistance, or repetitions over time to continually challenge the muscles and stimulate adaptation.

In addition to progressive overload, exercise variation is crucial to prevent plateaus and target different muscle fibers. By incorporating a variety of exercises into your program, you can ensure that all muscle groups are adequately stimulated and developed.

Balance and Proportion

When designing an upper body strengthening program, it is essential to strike a balance between different muscle groups. Overemphasizing certain muscle groups while neglecting others can lead to muscular imbalances and potential injuries.

Aim for a well-proportioned development of all major upper body muscle groups, including the chest, back, shoulders, arms, and core. This holistic approach ensures overall strength, functionality, and aesthetic appeal.

Warm-up and Cool-down

Proper warm-up and cool-down routines are integral components of any effective upper body strengthening program. A thorough warm-up prepares the body for exercise by elevating core temperature, increasing blood flow to the muscles, and enhancing flexibility.

A comprehensive cool-down routine promotes post-exercise recovery by reducing muscle soreness, promoting flexibility, and aiding in the removal of metabolic waste products.

Rest and Recovery

Adequate rest and recovery are paramount for muscle growth and regeneration. Allow ample time for rest between sets and exercises, and ensure sufficient sleep to facilitate the body's natural repair processes.

Listen to your body and take rest days when necessary. Overtraining can lead to burnout, decreased performance, and increased risk of injuries.

Conclusion

Comprehensive upper body strengthening requires a thoughtful combination of synergistic muscle group exercises, isolation exercises, progressive overload, exercise variation, and proper balance between different muscle groups. By adhering to these principles and incorporating adequate warm-up, cool-down, rest, and recovery into your program, you can effectively develop a strong, balanced, and well-defined upper body.

6.2 Increasing Difficulty and Intensity

The concept of increasing difficulty and intensity is a fundamental principle in various disciplines, particularly in the context of training and personal development. It refers to the gradual augmentation of challenges and demands placed on an individual or system, with the primary objective of promoting adaptation, growth, and improved performance.

Physiological Adaptations:

In the realm of physical training, increasing difficulty and intensity elicits specific physiological responses that drive adaptations and enhance fitness levels. As an individual engages in progressively challenging exercises, the body undergoes a series of biochemical and structural changes to meet the demands imposed. These adaptations include increased muscle mass and strength, improved cardiovascular capacity, and enhanced metabolic efficiency.

For instance, when an individual lifts heavier weights during resistance training, the muscles experience increased mechanical stress. In response, the body stimulates the synthesis of new muscle proteins, leading to muscle hypertrophy and increased strength. Similarly, when an individual runs at a faster pace or for longer distances, the cardiovascular system adapts by increasing the number and size of blood vessels and improving the efficiency of the heart.

Cognitive Adaptations:

Increasing difficulty and intensity also play a crucial role in cognitive development and learning. When individuals are exposed to challenging tasks that require sustained effort and focused attention, the brain undergoes a process of neuroplasticity. This involves the formation of new neural connections and the strengthening of existing ones, resulting in enhanced cognitive abilities.

For example, when a student engages in problem-solving exercises of increasing complexity, the brain areas responsible for logical reasoning, critical thinking, and memory are stimulated. Over time, the student develops a deeper understanding of the subject matter and improved problem-solving skills. Similarly, when a musician practices a challenging musical piece, the brain areas responsible for motor coordination, auditory processing, and musical expression are strengthened, leading to improved musical performance.

Psychological Adaptations:

In addition to physiological and cognitive adaptations, increasing difficulty and intensity can also foster psychological growth and resilience. When individuals face challenges and overcome them, they experience a sense of accomplishment and increased self-efficacy. This positive reinforcement can motivate them to continue pushing their limits and strive for excellence.

Moreover, exposure to challenging situations can help individuals develop coping mechanisms and learn to manage stress effectively. By facing adversity and learning from setbacks, they become more resilient and better equipped to handle future challenges. This psychological resilience is essential for personal growth and success in various aspects of life.

Principles of Gradual Progression:

It is important to note that the principle of increasing difficulty and intensity should be applied gradually and thoughtfully. Abrupt or excessive increases can lead to burnout, injury, or discouragement. Instead, challenges should be introduced incrementally, allowing the individual sufficient time to adapt and progress at a sustainable pace.

The rate of progression should be individualized, taking into account factors such as age, fitness level, and experience. Regular monitoring and assessment can help ensure that the level of difficulty and intensity is appropriate and aligns with the individual's goals and capabilities. By gradually exposing individuals to progressively challenging tasks, we stimulate physiological, cognitive, and psychological adaptations that enhance performance, promote growth, and build resilience. However, it is crucial to approach this principle with a thoughtful and gradual approach, ensuring that challenges are appropriate and allow for sustainable progress.

6.3 Mastering Balance and Control

In today's rapidly evolving business landscape, organizations face a relentless barrage of challenges that can disrupt operations, derail progress, and jeopardize stability. Amidst this turbulence, the ability to maintain balance and control has emerged as an essential survival skill for businesses that aspire to thrive.

Mastering balance and control requires a proactive and

multifaceted approach that encompasses strategic planning, operational resilience, and effective risk management. By embracing a proactive stance, organizations can anticipate potential disruptions, develop contingency plans, and implement safeguards to mitigate their impact. This foresight allows businesses to maintain stability, even in the face of unforeseen circumstances.

Operational resilience, a cornerstone of balance and control, ensures that businesses possess the adaptability and agility to withstand and recover from disruptions. This involves implementing robust business continuity plans, investing in technology infrastructure that supports remote work and collaboration, and fostering a culture of resilience among employees. By embracing operational resilience, organizations can minimize the impact of disruptions and ensure the smooth continuation of critical business functions.

Risk management, another vital aspect of balance and control, plays a pivotal role in mitigating the potential consequences of both internal and external threats. Organizations must establish a comprehensive risk management framework that identifies, assesses, and prioritizes risks, develops risk mitigation strategies, and monitors their effectiveness. By proactively managing risks, businesses can minimize the likelihood of disruptions and protect their financial, operational, and reputational well-being.

In addition to these core elements, mastering balance and control also requires a mindset shift from reactive to proactive management. Organizations must embrace a forward-looking perspective, continuously monitoring the business environment for potential disruptions and adapting their strategies accordingly. This proactive approach enables businesses to anticipate and address emerging challenges before they escalate into full-blown crises.

Furthermore, effective communication and collaboration are essential for maintaining balance and control. Organizations must foster open and transparent communication channels to keep all stakeholders informed about potential risks and disruptions, as well as the actions being taken to mitigate their impact. Collaboration across different departments and functions is also crucial to ensure a cohesive and coordinated response to challenges.

Mastering balance and control is not merely an abstract concept but a practical necessity for businesses navigating today's dynamic and unpredictable environment. By embracing strategic planning, operational resilience, and risk management, organizations can equip themselves with the tools and mindset necessary to weather storms, seize opportunities, and achieve sustained success.

Case Study: Navigating Disruption with Balance and Control

In the face of a global pandemic that forced businesses to adapt rapidly, ABC Corporation demonstrated the transformative power of balance and control. By leveraging its proactive planning, operational resilience, and robust risk management framework, ABC navigated the disruption with remarkable agility and resilience.

Prior to the pandemic, ABC had meticulously developed comprehensive business continuity plans that outlined detailed procedures for remote work, supply chain management, and customer support. These plans proved invaluable when the crisis hit, enabling ABC to transition seamlessly to remote operations and minimize disruptions to its supply chain and customer service.

In addition, ABC's investment in operational resilience paid off handsomely. The company had invested heavily in cloud-based technology infrastructure, which allowed its employees to work remotely without compromising productivity or collaboration. This investment ensured the continuity of critical business functions, even during periods of lockdown and social distancing.

Moreover, ABC's robust risk management framework played a key role in mitigating the financial and operational impact of the pandemic. The company had identified and assessed potential risks related to supply chain disruptions, travel restrictions, and employee absenteeism, and had developed contingency plans to address each of these risks. This foresight enabled ABC to respond swiftly to emerging challenges and minimize their impact on its business.

By proactively embracing balance and control, ABC Corporation was able to weather the storm of the pandemic and emerge stronger. The company's commitment to strategic planning, operational resilience, and risk management served as a beacon of stability amidst a sea of uncertainty, enabling it to continue serving its customers, protect its employees, and safeguard its financial well-being.

Best Practices for Mastering Balance and Control

Organizations seeking to master balance and control should consider the following best practices:

1. Develop a proactive mindset: Embrace a forward-looking perspective, continuously monitor the business environment, and anticipate potential disruptions.

2. Implement strategic planning: Establish clear goals and objectives, identify potential risks and opportunities, and develop plans to achieve your desired outcomes.
3. Build operational resilience: Invest in technology infrastructure, establish business continuity plans, and foster a culture of resilience among employees.
4. Implement a robust risk management framework: Identify, assess, prioritize, and mitigate potential risks to your organization.
5. Foster open and transparent communication: Keep stakeholders informed about potential risks and disruptions, and facilitate collaboration across departments and functions.
6. Continuously monitor and improve: Regularly evaluate your balance and control measures and make adjustments as needed to maintain alignment with your strategic objectives.

By adopting these best practices, organizations can lay the foundation for effective balance and control, empowering them to navigate the challenges of the 21st century business environment with confidence and resilience.

Chapter 7: Understanding Your Body's Feedback

7.1 Listening to Your Muscles

The human body is an incredibly complex and interconnected system, with each part playing a vital role in our overall health and well-being. Our muscles, in particular, are essential for movement, posture, and balance. They also play a key role in metabolism, energy production, and immune function.

As we go about our daily lives, our muscles constantly send us signals about their condition. These signals can be subtle, such as a slight ache or twinge, or they can be more pronounced, such as sharp pain or cramping. It is important to pay attention to these signals and to respond to them appropriately.

Ignoring muscle pain can lead to a number of problems, including:

Injury: If you continue to use a muscle that is in pain, you are more likely to injure it. This is because pain is a warning sign that the muscle is being overworked or damaged.
Chronic pain: Muscle pain that is not addressed can become chronic. This type of pain can be difficult to treat and can significantly impact your quality of life.
Reduced mobility: Muscle pain can make it difficult to

move around, which can lead to a loss of independence and a decreased quality of life.

How to Listen to Your Muscles

The first step to listening to your muscles is to be aware of how they feel. Pay attention to any aches, pains, or twinges that you experience. If you notice any pain, stop the activity that is causing it and rest the muscle.

If the pain is severe or does not go away after a few days, see a doctor. There may be an underlying medical condition that is causing the pain.

In addition to paying attention to pain, you can also listen to your muscles by:

Stretching: Stretching helps to keep muscles flexible and loose, which can help to prevent pain and injury.
Massage: Massage can help to relieve muscle tension and pain.
Heat and cold therapy: Heat can help to relax muscles, while cold can help to reduce inflammation and pain.
Exercise: Exercise can help to strengthen muscles and improve their endurance. However, it is important to listen to your body and stop if you experience any pain.

Benefits of Listening to Your Muscles

Listening to your muscles has a number of benefits, including:

Reduced pain: By listening to your muscles and responding to their signals, you can help to reduce pain and prevent injury.
Improved mobility: When your muscles are healthy and pain-free, you will be able to move more easily and with

greater range of motion.
Increased strength and endurance: Exercise can help to strengthen your muscles and improve their endurance. This can make it easier to perform everyday activities and participate in sports and other recreational activities.
Improved overall health and well-being: Healthy muscles are essential for overall health and well-being. They help to support the body, move the body, and produce energy.

Conclusion

Listening to your muscles is an important part of maintaining your health and well-being. By paying attention to the signals that your muscles send you, you can help to prevent pain, injury, and other problems. In addition, listening to your muscles can help you to improve your mobility, strength, endurance, and overall health.

7.2 Identifying and Correcting Form

Maintaining proper form is crucial in any physical activity, but especially in exercises that involve weights. Incorrect form can lead to injuries, decreased effectiveness of the exercise, and hinder progress. Identifying and correcting form is essential for maximizing the benefits of exercise while minimizing the risk of harm.

Identifying Form Errors

The first step in correcting form is identifying any errors. There are several common form errors that can occur during exercises, including:

- Incorrect posture: Maintaining a neutral spine and correct posture is crucial for preventing injuries and ensuring proper movement patterns.

- Improper grip: Using the wrong grip can strain muscles and joints, reducing the effectiveness of the exercise.
- Excessive range of motion: Going beyond the recommended range of motion can put unnecessary stress on joints and muscles, increasing the risk of injury.
- Incorrect breathing: Breathing correctly during exercises helps stabilize the body and improves performance. Incorrect breathing patterns can hinder progress and lead to discomfort.
- Unequal muscle activation: Using different muscle groups unevenly during an exercise can lead to imbalances, affecting performance and increasing the risk of injury.

Correcting Form Errors

Once form errors are identified, they must be corrected to ensure safe and effective exercise. The following steps can help improve form:

- Seek professional guidance: Consulting with a certified personal trainer or physical therapist can provide personalized guidance on proper form and ensure safe and effective exercise.
- Use mirrors and videos: Observing oneself in a mirror or recording videos of exercises can help identify form errors and make corrections accordingly.
- Focus on body awareness: Paying attention to body sensations during exercises can help identify areas where form may be incorrect.
- Use lighter weights: Starting with lighter weights allows for better control and focus on proper form. Gradually increase weight as form improves.
- Modify exercises: If an exercise is particularly challenging to perform with proper form, modify it to a variation that allows for correct movement patterns.

Benefits of Correct Form

Maintaining proper form during exercises offers numerous benefits, including:

- Injury prevention: Correct form reduces the risk of injuries by ensuring that joints and muscles are aligned and moving correctly.
- Increased effectiveness: Proper form allows for optimal muscle activation, maximizing the benefits of the exercise.
- Improved performance: Maintaining correct form enhances overall performance and progress in exercises.
- Reduced muscle imbalances: Correct form helps ensure that different muscle groups are activated evenly, reducing the risk of muscle imbalances.
- Enhanced body awareness: Focusing on proper form increases body awareness, improving coordination and overall movement quality.

Conclusion

Identifying and correcting form is essential for safe, effective, and beneficial exercises. By paying attention to body mechanics, using proper techniques, and seeking professional guidance when needed, individuals can minimize the risk of injuries, maximize the benefits of exercises, and achieve their fitness goals. Remember, proper form is not just about doing exercises correctly; it's about creating a foundation for lifelong healthy movement patterns.

7.3 Preventing Injuries and Overtraining

Maintaining a healthy and active lifestyle through exercise is paramount for overall well-being. However, it is essential to approach fitness with caution to prevent injuries and overtraining. Overexertion can lead to a myriad of physical setbacks that can hinder progress and even jeopardize long-term health goals. Therefore, it is crucial to implement preventative measures and adhere to guidelines to safeguard your body from harm.

Injury Prevention

Injuries are a common occurrence in the realm of physical activity. They can range in severity from minor sprains and strains to more debilitating fractures and dislocations. To minimize the risk of injury, it is imperative to follow these fundamental principles:

1. Warm-up and Cool-down:

Prior to any exercise session, dedicate a few minutes to warm up your muscles. This prepares the body for the exertion to come, enhancing flexibility and reducing the likelihood of strains or tears. Similarly, after your workout, allow time for a cool-down period to gradually lower your heart rate and facilitate muscle recovery.

2. Proper Technique:

Mastering the correct form for each exercise is vital. Incorrect technique can put undue stress on certain muscles or joints, increasing the risk of injury. If unsure about proper form, seek guidance from a qualified fitness professional.

3. Gradual Progression:

Avoid pushing yourself too hard too soon. Gradually increase the intensity and duration of your workouts to allow your body to adapt and strengthen. Overexertion can lead to injuries, burnout, and decreased motivation.

4. Rest and Recovery:

Adequate rest is crucial for muscle repair and recovery. Incorporate rest days into your training schedule to prevent cumulative fatigue and promote optimal performance. Ignoring the need for rest can compromise your immune system and increase susceptibility to injury.

5. Listen to Your Body:

Pay attention to how your body responds to exercise. If you experience any pain or discomfort, stop the activity and seek professional advice. Pushing through pain can worsen injuries and prolong recovery time.

Overtraining

Overtraining is a condition that arises when the body is subjected to excessive physical exertion without sufficient rest. It can manifest in a variety of symptoms, including:

1. Physical Signs:

- Chronic muscle soreness
- Fatigue and lack of energy
- Decreased performance
- Increased susceptibility to injury
- Sleep disturbances

2. Emotional Symptoms:

- Irritability and mood swings
- Loss of motivation
- Difficulty concentrating
- Anxiety

To prevent overtraining, it is essential to:

1. Monitor Your Workouts:

Keep a training log to track your exercise intensity, duration, and frequency. This will help you identify patterns and avoid overexertion.

2. Incorporate Variety:

Engage in different types of exercises to work various muscle groups. This will prevent overuse injuries and promote overall fitness.

3. Listen to Your Body:

As mentioned earlier, pay attention to your body's signals. If you experience any symptoms of overtraining, take a break and allow yourself time to recover.

4. Prioritize Sleep:

Sleep is essential for muscle recovery and overall well-being. Aim for 7-9 hours of quality sleep each night.

5. Fuel Your Body:

Provide your body with adequate nutrition to support your training demands. Consume a balanced diet that includes plenty of protein, carbohydrates, and healthy fats.

Conclusion

Injury prevention and avoiding overtraining are crucial aspects of maintaining a healthy and sustainable fitness routine. By implementing the strategies outlined above, you can minimize the risk of setbacks and maximize your progress towards your fitness goals. Remember to listen to your body, warm up and cool down properly, follow proper technique, progress gradually, and incorporate rest and recovery into your training schedule. By prioritizing these principles, you can enjoy the benefits of exercise while safeguarding your physical well-being.

Chapter 8: Adapting Workouts for Different Levels

8.1 Modifying Exercises for Beginners

Embarking on a fitness journey can be daunting, especially for beginners who may face limitations or discomfort with certain exercises. To ensure a safe and effective workout experience, it is essential to modify exercises to accommodate individual needs and abilities. Exercise modifications can reduce strain on joints, minimize risk of injury, and improve form, ultimately enhancing the overall fitness experience.

Principles of Exercise Modification

When modifying exercises, several principles should be considered:

Gradual Progression: Begin with exercises that are manageable and gradually increase intensity and complexity as strength and endurance improve.
Range of Motion: Ensure that the range of motion is appropriate for the individual's flexibility and mobility. Avoid overstretching or straining joints.
Joint Stability: Focus on exercises that provide stability to joints, preventing excessive movement that could lead to injury.
Muscle Activation: Choose exercises that effectively engage target muscles without overtaxing them.

Proper Form: Maintain correct body alignment and technique throughout the exercise to minimize risk of strain or injury.

Exercise Modification Techniques

Numerous techniques can be employed to modify exercises for beginners:

Reduce Weight: Begin with lighter weights or no weight at all. Gradually increase resistance as strength develops.
Alter Repetition Range: Start with fewer repetitions and gradually increase the number as endurance improves.
Shorten Range of Motion: Modify exercises to target a smaller range of motion until flexibility and mobility improve.
Use Assist Devices: Utilize resistance bands, stability balls, or other assistive devices to support and stabilize movements.
Modify Exercise Type: Substitute exercises with lower impact or reduced joint strain, such as squats instead of lunges or swimming instead of running.
Break Down Movements: Divide complex exercises into smaller, simpler components to enhance technique and focus on specific muscle groups.
Use Bodyweight: Leverage bodyweight exercises like push-ups and squats to build strength without external resistance.

Benefits of Exercise Modification

Modifying exercises offers numerous benefits for beginners:

Injury Prevention: Reduced risk of strain, sprains, and other injuries by accommodating individual limitations.
Improved Form: Focus on proper technique and alignment,

preventing compensation patterns that could lead to pain or discomfort.
Increased Confidence: Encourages beginners to engage in physical activity without feeling overwhelmed or discouraged.
Enhanced Enjoyment: Makes exercise more enjoyable and sustainable by reducing discomfort and increasing effectiveness.
Long-Term Progress: Facilitates gradual progression to more challenging exercises, supporting consistent fitness development.

Consulting with a Professional

For personalized exercise modifications, it is highly recommended to consult with a qualified healthcare professional, such as a physical therapist, exercise physiologist, or certified personal trainer. These experts can assess individual needs, recommend appropriate modifications, and provide guidance on safe and effective exercise practices.

Conclusion

Modifying exercises for beginners is crucial to ensure a safe, enjoyable, and effective fitness experience. By adhering to the principles of modification and employing various techniques, individuals can customize their workouts to their current abilities and gradually progress towards their fitness goals. Consulting with a qualified professional can provide further support and ensure optimal exercise modifications that address individual needs.

8.2 Progressing to Intermediate and Advanced Levels

As you progress in your learning journey, you will encounter increasingly complex language and grammar structures. This section will provide you with strategies and techniques to effectively navigate intermediate and advanced levels of language proficiency.

Expanding Vocabulary and Grammar

At intermediate levels, your vocabulary should encompass a wide range of topics and domains. Focus on acquiring words that are commonly used in everyday conversations, academic settings, and professional contexts. Engage with authentic materials such as books, articles, and movies to encounter unfamiliar words in meaningful contexts. Additionally, utilize dictionaries and online resources to explore the nuances and connotations of new words.

Grammar proficiency is crucial for expressing yourself accurately and fluently. Study advanced grammar structures, including conditionals, modals, and passive voice. Practice using them in different contexts to gain confidence and accuracy. Seek feedback from native speakers or language teachers to refine your usage.

Developing Fluency and Accuracy

Fluency refers to the ability to speak or write smoothly and effortlessly. Engage in regular speaking practice with native speakers or language partners. Focus on producing sentences that are grammatically correct and convey your intended meaning clearly. Don't be afraid to make mistakes; they are an essential part of the learning process.

Accuracy involves using the correct vocabulary and grammar. Utilize dictionaries, grammar guides, and language learning apps to ensure that your language use is precise. Pay attention to the details, such as verb tenses, prepositions, and articles. Regular writing practice can also help improve your accuracy.

Understanding Cultural Context

Language is deeply intertwined with culture. To fully understand a language, it is essential to immerse yourself in its cultural context. Read literature, watch movies, and interact with native speakers from the target language country. Participate in cultural events and customs to gain insights into the nuances of the language and its speakers.

Setting Goals and Monitoring Progress

Establish clear goals for your intermediate and advanced learning. Determine the specific areas you want to improve, such as fluency, accuracy, or cultural understanding. Monitor your progress regularly by tracking your vocabulary growth, grammar mastery, and overall confidence in speaking and writing. Seek feedback from others to identify areas for improvement.

Maintaining Motivation and Perseverance

Learning a language at intermediate and advanced levels requires dedication and perseverance. Set realistic expectations and avoid feeling overwhelmed. Break down your learning into manageable chunks and celebrate your successes along the way. Find ways to make learning enjoyable by incorporating it into your hobbies or interests.

Conclusion

Progressing to intermediate and advanced levels of language proficiency requires a comprehensive approach that encompasses vocabulary expansion, grammar mastery, fluency development, accuracy, cultural understanding, goal setting, and motivation. By implementing these strategies, you can effectively navigate the complexities of advanced language use and achieve your language learning goals.

8.3 Finding the Right Challenge for Your Fitness Level

Before embarking on any fitness program, it is crucial to assess your current fitness level. This will help you determine the appropriate intensity and duration of your workouts, minimizing the risk of injury and maximizing results. Several methods can be used to assess fitness, including:

Cardiovascular endurance: Measured by activities that increase your heart rate, such as running, cycling, or swimming. Common tests include the 12-minute run test or the VO2 max test.
Muscular strength: Measured by your ability to exert force against resistance. Tests include bench press, leg press, or pull-ups.
Muscular endurance: Measured by how long you can sustain muscular effort. Tests include push-ups, planks, or squats.
Flexibility: Measured by your range of motion in joints. Tests include the sit-and-reach test or the shoulder stretch test.

Choosing the Right Challenge

Once you have assessed your fitness level, you can start selecting exercises and activities that provide an appropriate challenge. Here are some guidelines:

Beginner: Start with exercises that are easy to perform, gradually increasing the intensity and duration as you progress. Focus on establishing a consistent exercise routine before pushing yourself too hard.
Intermediate: Aim for exercises that challenge you but still allow you to maintain good form. Include variations and progressions to keep your workouts interesting and effective.
Advanced: Choose exercises that require significant strength, endurance, or flexibility. Incorporate advanced techniques such as compound exercises, plyometrics, or high-intensity interval training (HIIT).

Finding the Optimal Challenge

The optimal challenge will vary depending on your fitness goals, current fitness level, and personal preferences. It should be challenging enough to push you out of your comfort zone but not so difficult that it becomes overwhelming or discourages you. Here are some tips for finding the right balance:

Listen to your body: Pay attention to how you feel during and after workouts. If you experience excessive fatigue, soreness, or pain, it may be a sign that you need to reduce the intensity or duration.
Set realistic goals: Don't try to achieve too much too soon. Start with small, achievable goals and gradually increase the challenge as you progress.
Experiment with different exercises: Find activities that you enjoy and challenge you physically. Variety can help prevent boredom and keep you motivated.
Seek professional guidance: If you are unsure about the right challenge for you, consult with a certified personal trainer or other qualified fitness professional.

Progression and Adjustment

As you progress in your fitness journey, it is important to adjust the challenge accordingly. If workouts become too easy, it's time to increase the intensity or duration. If you experience difficulty maintaining good form or recovering adequately, consider reducing the challenge. Regular assessments can help you track your progress and make necessary adjustments to stay on track towards your fitness goals.

Remember: The goal is to find a challenge that promotes growth, prevents stagnation, and ultimately leads to a healthier and more fulfilling life.

Chapter 9: Incorporating Wall Workouts into Your Routine

9.1 Building a Weekly Training Schedule

A well-structured weekly training schedule is paramount for achieving your fitness goals effectively and efficiently. Whether you're a seasoned athlete or just starting out, creating a plan that aligns with your specific needs and abilities is crucial. Here are some key considerations and steps to guide you in building a tailored weekly training schedule:

1. Determine Your Goals:

Start by clearly defining your fitness objectives. Are you aiming to improve endurance, gain strength, lose weight, or enhance overall athleticism. Identifying your goals will help you prioritize activities and allocate training time accordingly.

2. Assess Your Fitness Level:

Take stock of your current fitness level to establish a realistic starting point. Consider your cardiovascular endurance, muscular strength, and flexibility. This assessment will guide you in selecting appropriate exercises and intensities.

3. Choose Activities You Enjoy:

Exercise should be enjoyable, not a chore. Select activities that you genuinely find engaging. This will increase your motivation and make it more likely that you'll stick to your schedule.

4. Include a Variety of Exercises:

Incorporate a range of exercises into your plan to target different muscle groups and fitness components. This will prevent boredom, promote balanced development, and minimize the risk of overuse injuries.

5. Structure Your Week:

Determine how many days per week you can dedicate to training. Divide your activities into appropriate sessions, ensuring rest and recovery days. Plan for strength training, cardiovascular exercise, and flexibility work as needed.

6. Set Realistic Goals:

Avoid setting overly ambitious goals that could lead to burnout or injury. Start with achievable targets and gradually increase intensity and duration as your fitness progresses.

7. Include Warm-Ups and Cool-Downs:

Always begin your workouts with a light warm-up to prepare your body for exercise. Similarly, end each session with a cool-down to reduce muscle soreness and improve flexibility.

8. Listen to Your Body:

Pay attention to how your body responds to training. If you

experience pain or discomfort, adjust your routine or consult with a medical professional. Rest is an integral part of the training process, allowing your body to repair and rebuild.

Sample Weekly Training Schedule:

The following is an example of a weekly training schedule for someone with intermediate fitness levels:

Monday: Strength training (upper body), cardiovascular exercise (45 minutes)
Tuesday: Rest
Wednesday: Strength training (lower body), flexibility work (20 minutes)
Thursday: Cardiovascular exercise (30 minutes)
Friday: Strength training (full body)
Saturday: Active recovery (e.g., hiking, swimming)
Sunday: Rest

Remember, this is just a sample schedule. Adjust it based on your individual needs and preferences. Consistency is key, so find a routine that you can stick to over time.

9.2 Integrating Wall Workouts with Other Forms of Exercise

Wall workouts, with their versatility and adaptability, can be seamlessly integrated into any fitness regimen, complementing other forms of exercise and enhancing overall fitness goals. Here's how to effectively combine wall workouts with other modalities:

Resistance Training:

Wall workouts provide an excellent foundation for

resistance training, particularly for compound movements that engage multiple muscle groups simultaneously. Wall squats, push-ups, and rows target major muscle groups, fostering strength and muscle development. These exercises can be modified to suit various fitness levels, from beginners to advanced athletes.

Integrating wall workouts into a resistance training routine can enhance muscle activation and recruitment. By utilizing the wall as a stable and supportive surface, individuals can focus on proper form and execution, reducing the risk of injury and maximizing training effectiveness. Wall workouts can also be incorporated as warm-ups or cool-downs, preparing the body for more intense resistance exercises or aiding in post-workout recovery.

Cardiovascular Exercise:

Wall workouts can also complement cardiovascular exercise, providing a low-impact and effective way to elevate heart rate and burn calories. High-intensity interval training (HIIT) workouts, characterized by alternating bursts of high-intensity exercise with brief recovery periods, can be effectively performed using wall-based exercises. Wall jumps, burpees, and mountain climbers engage large muscle groups and challenge the cardiovascular system.

By incorporating wall workouts into a cardio routine, individuals can diversify their training and minimize repetitive stress on joints and muscles. Wall exercises offer a unique and challenging approach to cardiovascular training, making it more enjoyable and engaging.

Flexibility and Mobility:

Wall workouts can enhance flexibility and mobility by stretching and lengthening muscles. Wall stretches, such as calf stretches, hamstring stretches, and quad stretches, effectively target specific muscle groups and improve range of motion. By utilizing the wall as support and leverage, individuals can deepen stretches and improve posture.

Integrating wall stretches into a regular exercise routine can help reduce muscle tightness, improve joint mobility, and enhance overall flexibility. Regular stretching promotes relaxation, reduces the risk of injuries, and supports optimal physical performance.

Balance and Stability:

Wall workouts can also improve balance and stability by engaging core muscles and enhancing proprioception (body awareness). Exercises like wall sits, single-leg wall squats, and toe taps challenge balance and stability, strengthening the muscles responsible for maintaining upright posture and coordination.

Incorporating wall workouts into a balance and stability routine can benefit individuals of all ages and fitness levels. Improved balance and stability reduce the risk of falls, enhance athletic performance, and support everyday activities.

Tailoring the Integration:

The integration of wall workouts with other forms of exercise should be tailored to individual fitness goals and abilities. Beginners may start by incorporating wall exercises into their warm-ups or cool-downs, gradually increasing intensity and duration as they progress. Advanced athletes can incorporate wall workouts into their resistance training, cardio routines, and flexibility sessions to enhance overall performance and fitness.

It is crucial to listen to your body and rest when needed. Proper hydration and nutrition are essential for optimal recovery and training outcomes. Consultation with a qualified fitness professional can provide personalized guidance on integrating wall workouts effectively and safely. By integrating wall exercises into resistance training, cardiovascular exercise, flexibility and mobility routines, and balance and stability programs, individuals can optimize their training, reduce the risk of injuries, and enjoy a well-rounded fitness experience. With proper integration, wall workouts can contribute significantly to achieving desired fitness outcomes, whether they involve building strength, improving endurance, enhancing flexibility, or maintaining balance.

9.3 Tips for Consistency and Motivation

Maintaining consistency and motivation is crucial for achieving any goal, whether it's completing a degree, losing weight, or starting a new business. However, it can be challenging to stay on track, especially when faced with setbacks or periods of low motivation. Here are nine tips to help you overcome these challenges and stay consistent with your goals:

1. Set Realistic Goals:

One of the biggest reasons people fail to achieve their goals is that they set unrealistic expectations. If your goals are too ambitious, you're likely to get discouraged and give up. Instead, start with small, achievable goals that you can gradually build upon. As you make progress, you'll gain confidence and momentum, which will make it easier to stay motivated.

2. Break Down Tasks into Smaller Steps:

If you have a large or complex goal, it can be overwhelming to think about how you're going to achieve it. Break the task down into smaller, more manageable steps. This will make it seem less daunting and help you stay focused on the present moment.

3. Create a Plan:

Once you have your goals and steps outlined, create a plan for how you're going to achieve them. This plan should include specific actions, deadlines, and resources. Having a plan will give you a sense of direction and help you stay on track.

4. Find an Accountability Partner:

Having someone to hold you accountable can be a great way to stay motivated. Find a friend, family member, or colleague who is also working towards a goal. Check in with each other regularly to share progress, offer support, and hold each other accountable.

5. Reward Yourself:

When you achieve a milestone, no matter how small, take the time to reward yourself. This will help you stay motivated and make the process more enjoyable. Rewards can be anything that you enjoy, such as buying yourself a new book, going out to dinner, or taking a break from work.

6. Visualize Success:

Take some time each day to visualize yourself achieving your goals. See yourself crossing the finish line, receiving your diploma, or starting your own business. This will help you stay focused and motivated, even when things get tough.

7. Positive Self-Talk:

Pay attention to the way you talk to yourself. If you're constantly putting yourself down, you're going to have a hard time staying motivated. Instead, focus on positive self-talk. Tell yourself that you can do it, that you're strong, and that you're capable of achieving anything you set your mind to.

8. Don't Be Afraid to Ask for Help:

If you're struggling to stay consistent and motivated, don't be afraid to ask for help. Talk to a friend, family member, therapist, or coach. They can provide support, encouragement, and advice.

9. Remember Your Why:

When you're feeling discouraged, take some time to think about why you started working towards your goals in the first place. What are you hoping to achieve. How will achieving your goals make your life better. Keep your why in mind, and it will help you stay motivated even when things get tough.

Chapter 10: Nutrition for Upper Body Strength

10.1 Understanding Macronutrients

Macronutrients are the essential nutrients that the body requires in large amounts to function properly. They are classified into three main groups: carbohydrates, proteins, and fats. Each macronutrient plays a specific role in the body and provides different types of energy.

Carbohydrates

Carbohydrates are the body's primary source of energy. They are broken down into glucose, which is then used by the body for energy. Carbohydrates are found in a variety of foods, including bread, pasta, rice, fruits, and vegetables.

Proteins

Proteins are essential for building and repairing tissues. They are also involved in a variety of other bodily functions, such as hormone production and immune function. Proteins are found in a variety of foods, including meat, poultry, fish, eggs, and dairy products.

Fats

Fats are an important source of energy and they also help

to protect the body's organs. Fats are found in a variety of foods, including butter, margarine, oil, nuts, and seeds.

The Importance of Macronutrients

Macronutrients are essential for good health. They provide the body with the energy and nutrients it needs to function properly. Eating a balanced diet that includes all three macronutrients is important for maintaining a healthy weight and reducing the risk of chronic diseases.

Recommended Daily Intake of Macronutrients

The recommended daily intake of macronutrients varies depending on age, sex, and activity level. However, the following general guidelines can be used:

Carbohydrates: 45-65% of total calories
Proteins: 10-35% of total calories
Fats: 20-35% of total calories

Choosing Healthy Macronutrient Sources

When choosing foods to meet your macronutrient needs, it is important to choose healthy sources. For example, whole grains are a better source of carbohydrates than refined grains. Lean protein sources, such as chicken and fish, are better than fatty protein sources, such as red meat. Healthy fats, such as olive oil and avocados, are better than unhealthy fats, such as saturated and trans fats.

Supplements

In some cases, it may be necessary to take supplements to meet your macronutrient needs. For example, athletes may need to take protein supplements to support their muscle growth and recovery. However, it is important to talk to a doctor before taking any supplements.

Conclusion

Macronutrients are essential for good health. Eating a balanced diet that includes all three macronutrients is important for maintaining a healthy weight and reducing the risk of chronic diseases. When choosing foods to meet your macronutrient needs, it is important to choose healthy sources. In some cases, it may be necessary to take supplements to meet your macronutrient needs. However, it is important to talk to a doctor before taking any supplements.

10.2 Fueling Your Workouts

Introduction

Proper nutrition plays a crucial role in optimizing performance and recovery during workouts. Understanding the principles of sports nutrition empowers individuals to make informed dietary choices that support their fitness goals. This one delves into the fundamental aspects of fueling workouts, providing a comprehensive guide to optimizing nutrient intake before, during, and after exercise.

Pre-Workout Nutrition

The primary objective of pre-workout nutrition is to provide the body with the energy and nutrients it needs to perform at its best. Carbohydrates serve as the main source of fuel, as they are readily broken down into glucose, the body's primary energy source. Complex carbohydrates, such as whole grains, fruits, and vegetables, provide sustained energy release over time.

Protein is also essential for pre-workout nutrition, as it helps maintain muscle mass and supports tissue repair. A combination of carbohydrates and protein consumed 1-2 hours before exercise is recommended for optimal performance.

Intra-Workout Nutrition

During prolonged or intense workouts, the body's glycogen stores may become depleted, leading to fatigue and impaired performance. Consuming carbohydrates during exercise can help replenish glycogen levels and maintain blood sugar levels. Sports drinks, energy gels, or fruit can be effective ways to provide carbohydrates during workouts. The timing and amount of intra-workout carbohydrates depend on the intensity and duration of exercise.

Post-Workout Nutrition

The primary goal of post-workout nutrition is to promote muscle recovery and replenish glycogen stores. Protein is essential for muscle repair and growth, and should be consumed within 30-60 minutes after exercise. Carbohydrates are also important for replenishing glycogen levels and providing energy for recovery processes. A combination of protein and carbohydrates in a ratio of approximately 3:1 is recommended for optimal post-workout recovery.

Hydration

Hydration is essential for optimal performance and recovery. Dehydration can lead to fatigue, impaired cognitive function, and increased risk of injury. It is important to consume fluids before, during, and after exercise to maintain adequate hydration levels. Water is the most effective choice for hydration, but sports drinks can be beneficial for prolonged or intense workouts, as they provide carbohydrates and electrolytes.

Supplements

While a well-rounded diet can provide the necessary nutrients for fueling workouts, certain supplements may provide additional benefits. Creatine, for example, has been shown to improve muscle strength and power. Beta-alanine can enhance endurance performance by buffering lactic acid. Caffeine can stimulate the central nervous system, providing a boost in energy and focus. It is important to consult with a healthcare professional before taking any supplements to ensure safety and effectiveness.

Individualized Approach

Optimal nutrition for fueling workouts varies depending on individual factors such as body size, fitness level, and exercise type. It is essential to experiment with different nutrition strategies to determine what works best for each person. Monitoring progress and making adjustments as needed is key to optimizing performance and recovery.

Conclusion

Fueling workouts effectively requires a comprehensive approach that considers pre-, intra-, and post-workout nutrition, as well as hydration and supplementation strategies. By understanding the principles of sports nutrition, individuals can make informed dietary choices that support their fitness goals, enhance performance, and promote recovery. Remember that consistency and personalization are key to maximizing the benefits of nutrition for workouts.

10.3 Supplementing for Optimal Results

In today's fast-paced world, it can be challenging to maintain a healthy diet that provides all the essential nutrients our bodies need. Supplements can play a valuable role in bridging the gap between our dietary intake and optimal nutrient levels. However, it's crucial to approach supplementation with a balanced and informed approach to maximize benefits while minimizing risks.

The Role of Supplements

Supplements are products that contain concentrated forms of vitamins, minerals, herbs, or other substances intended to enhance nutrient intake. They come in various forms, including tablets, capsules, powders, and liquids. Supplements can be beneficial for individuals who:

Have difficulty meeting nutrient requirements through diet alone
Experience nutrient deficiencies or imbalances
Are at risk for specific health conditions
Want to support overall well-being

Choosing the Right Supplements

The key to effective supplementation is choosing the right products for your individual needs. Consider the following factors:

Nutrient Deficiencies: Identify any nutrient deficiencies through blood tests or dietary analysis and choose supplements that target those specific nutrients.
Health Conditions: Some supplements can support specific health conditions, such as glucosamine for joint health or omega-3 fatty acids for heart health.
Quality and Safety: Choose supplements from reputable

manufacturers that adhere to industry standards and undergo rigorous testing.

Dosage and Frequency

The recommended dosage and frequency of supplementation vary depending on the nutrient and individual factors. Always follow the instructions on the supplement label or consult a healthcare professional for personalized guidance. It's important to avoid excessive supplementation, as it can lead to adverse effects.

Types of Supplements

The wide range of available supplements can be classified into several categories:

Vitamins: Essential organic compounds that the body cannot produce on its own.
Minerals: Inorganic elements that play vital roles in various bodily functions.
Herbs and Botanicals: Plant-derived substances with medicinal properties.
Other Supplements: Products such as probiotics, amino acids, and enzymes that support specific aspects of health.

Interactions and Side Effects

Supplements can interact with certain medications or other supplements. It's essential to disclose all supplements you are taking to your healthcare provider to avoid potential adverse reactions. Side effects of supplementation can vary depending on the nutrient, dosage, and individual sensitivity. Always read the supplement label carefully and consult a healthcare professional if you experience any adverse reactions.

Informed Supplementation

Supplementation should be an informed decision based on individual needs and potential benefits and risks. By following these guidelines, you can use supplements to enhance your nutrient intake, support overall well-being, and optimize your health outcomes:

Consult with a healthcare professional before starting any supplementation.
Choose high-quality supplements from reputable manufacturers.
Determine your individual nutrient needs and target specific deficiencies.
Follow the recommended dosage and frequency guidelines.
Monitor your response to supplementation and report any adverse reactions to your healthcare provider.
Consider the potential interactions between supplements and medications.

Remember, supplementation is not a substitute for a balanced diet. Focus on consuming whole, nutrient-rich foods as the foundation of your health. Supplements can complement a healthy lifestyle and support your body's optimal functioning.

Chapter 11: Rest and Recovery

11.1 Importance of Rest Days

In the relentless pursuit of fitness goals, the allure of pushing ourselves to the brink can be intoxicating. However, amidst the rigorous training regimen, it is crucial to recognize the paramount importance of rest days. While exercise is undoubtedly a cornerstone of physical well-being, neglecting adequate rest can not only hinder progress but also lead to detrimental consequences.

Physiological Recovery and Adaptation

During intense exercise, our muscles undergo microscopic tears. Rest days provide the necessary time for these tears to repair and rebuild, leading to increased muscle strength and endurance. Furthermore, rest allows the body to replenish glycogen stores, the primary fuel source for high-intensity activities. Without sufficient rest, muscles remain in a weakened state, impairing performance and increasing the risk of injury.

Hormonal Balance

Exercise triggers the release of hormones such as cortisol, which plays a role in energy regulation and stress response. While cortisol is essential for short-term performance, chronic elevations due to inadequate rest can suppress the immune system, hinder muscle recovery, and increase the risk of overtraining syndrome. Rest days allow cortisol levels to return to baseline, promoting optimal hormonal balance and reducing the likelihood of hormonal dysregulation.

Mental and Emotional Well-being

Exercise exerts a profound impact on mental and emotional health, reducing stress, improving mood, and enhancing cognitive function. However, excessive exercise without sufficient rest can lead to burnout, irritability, and anxiety. Rest days provide an opportunity for psychological rejuvenation, allowing us to recharge our batteries and return to training with renewed vigor and enthusiasm.

Injury Prevention

Pushing through fatigue and neglecting rest days can increase the risk of acute injuries such as muscle strains, sprains, and fractures. Overuse injuries, such as tendinitis and stress fractures, can also develop insidiously due to chronic lack of rest. By incorporating rest days into our training schedule, we allow our bodies to recover adequately, reducing the strain on muscles, joints, and connective tissues, and minimizing the likelihood of injury.

Optimal Performance and Long-term Gains

Rest days are not simply periods of inactivity but rather an integral part of an effective fitness regimen. By allowing our bodies to recover and rebuild, we set the stage for optimal performance in subsequent workouts. Neglecting rest days may provide short-term gratification but can ultimately lead to plateaus or even setbacks in our fitness journey. Consistent adherence to a training schedule that includes rest days maximizes long-term progress and reduces the risk of burnout and injuries.

Conclusion

Rest days are an indispensable component of any well-rounded fitness plan. By providing our bodies with the time they need to recover, adapt, and rejuvenate, we optimize our physical, mental, and emotional well-being. Incorporating rest days into our training schedule is not a sign of weakness but rather a strategic investment in our long-term fitness goals. By embracing the importance of rest, we unlock the full potential of our bodies and minds, paving the way for sustained progress and a healthier, more fulfilling life.

11.2 Techniques for Muscle Recovery

Exercise is an essential part of a healthy lifestyle, but it can also lead to muscle soreness and fatigue. This is especially true if you're new to exercise or if you're pushing yourself harder than usual. Muscle recovery is the process of repairing and rebuilding muscle tissue after exercise. It's an important part of the training process, and it can help you to improve your performance and reduce your risk of injury.

There are a number of different techniques that you can use to speed up muscle recovery. Some of the most effective include:

1. Active recovery

Active recovery involves doing light exercise after a workout. This helps to increase blood flow to the muscles, which can help to remove waste products and speed up the repair process. Some good examples of active recovery activities include walking, swimming, or biking.

2. Static stretching

Static stretching involves holding a stretch for 20-30 seconds. This helps to improve flexibility and range of motion, which can reduce muscle soreness and stiffness. Some good examples of static stretches include the quadriceps stretch, the hamstring stretch, and the calf stretch.

3. Foam rolling

Foam rolling is a type of self-massage that can help to release muscle tension and improve blood flow. It's a great way to relieve muscle soreness and stiffness.

4. Massage

Massage is another great way to relieve muscle soreness and stiffness. It helps to increase blood flow and lymphatic drainage, which can help to remove waste products and speed up the repair process.

5. Cold therapy

Cold therapy can help to reduce inflammation and muscle soreness. It can be applied to the affected area in the form of an ice pack or a cold bath.

6. Heat therapy

Heat therapy can help to relax muscles and relieve pain. It can be applied to the affected area in the form of a heating pad or a hot bath.

7. Nutrition

Eating a healthy diet is important for overall health and well-being, but it's also important for muscle recovery. Make sure to eat plenty of protein, carbohydrates, and healthy fats. Protein is essential for repairing and rebuilding muscle tissue, carbohydrates provide energy, and healthy fats help to reduce inflammation.

8. Sleep

Sleep is essential for muscle recovery. When you sleep, your body releases hormones that help to repair and rebuild muscle tissue. Make sure to get 7-8 hours of sleep each night.

9. Hydration

Staying hydrated is important for overall health and well-being, but it's also important for muscle recovery. Dehydration can lead to muscle cramps and soreness. Make sure to drink plenty of fluids throughout the day, especially before, during, and after exercise.

10. Rest

Rest is an important part of the muscle recovery process. It gives your body time to repair and rebuild muscle tissue. Make sure to take a day or two off from exercise each week to allow your muscles to recover.

By following these tips, you can speed up muscle recovery and improve your performance. Remember, muscle recovery is an important part of the training process, and it's essential for preventing injury and maximizing your results.

11.3 Recognizing Signs of Overtraining

Overtraining occurs when an individual engages in excessive exercise without allowing for adequate rest and recovery, resulting in a state of physical and mental exhaustion. Recognizing the signs of overtraining is crucial for athletes, fitness enthusiasts, and healthcare professionals alike to prevent potential health risks and optimize performance.

Physical Signs:

Persistent Fatigue: Overtraining can lead to unrelenting fatigue that persists even after rest.
Reduced Performance: A significant decrease in performance despite maintaining or increasing training intensity may indicate overtraining.
Muscle Soreness and Pain: Muscles remain sore and painful even after extended periods of rest.
Increased Resting Heart Rate: The heart rate remains elevated even during rest or light activity.
Sleep Disturbances: Overtraining can disrupt sleep patterns, leading to difficulty falling or staying asleep.
Gastrointestinal Distress: Nausea, vomiting, and diarrhea can be symptoms of overtraining.
Weight Loss or Gain: Unintended weight loss or gain may be a sign of overtraining.
Increased Susceptibility to Illness: Overtraining can weaken the immune system, making individuals more prone to infections.
Hormonal Imbalances: Overtraining can disrupt hormone production, leading to changes in menstrual cycles, mood swings, and loss of appetite.

Mental and Emotional Signs:

Mood Changes: Irritability, mood swings, and depression can be indicative of overtraining.
Lack of Motivation: Loss of interest or motivation for

training activities may suggest overtraining.
Difficulty Concentrating: Cognitive function can be impaired due to overtraining.
Increased Anxiety: Overtraining can lead to heightened anxiety levels.
Emotional Instability: Emotional outbursts, crying spells, or feelings of hopelessness can be signs of overtraining.
Withdrawal from Social Activities: Individuals experiencing overtraining may withdraw from social interactions and hobbies.

Other Signs:

Elevated Creatine Kinase Levels: Blood tests may reveal elevated levels of creatine kinase, an enzyme released from damaged muscle cells.
Suppressed Immune Function: Overtraining can impair immune cell function, making individuals more susceptible to illness.
Electrolyte Imbalances: Excessive sweating during training can lead to electrolyte imbalances, causing fatigue and muscle cramps.
Cardiovascular Dysfunction: Overtraining can strain the cardiovascular system, resulting in palpitations or shortness of breath.

It is important to note that some of these signs can also be associated with other medical conditions. Therefore, it is essential to consult a healthcare professional for a thorough evaluation and diagnosis if experiencing any of the aforementioned symptoms.

Addressing Overtraining:

If overtraining is suspected, it is crucial to take immediate action to prevent further health complications. Rest is the primary remedy for overtraining. Gradually reduce training intensity and duration until symptoms subside. Adequate sleep, nutrition, and hydration are also essential for recovery.

Mental health support may be necessary to address the emotional and psychological toll of overtraining. Therapy or counseling can provide coping mechanisms and strategies for managing stress and anxiety.

Prevention Strategies:

To prevent overtraining, follow these guidelines:

Listen to Your Body: Pay attention to your body's signals and take rest days when needed.
Gradual Progression: Gradually increase training intensity and duration over time to avoid overwhelming the body.
Periodization: Plan training programs with periods of high intensity followed by periods of rest and recovery.
Cross-Training: Incorporate different activities into your routine to reduce stress on specific muscle groups.
Adequate Nutrition: Consume a balanced diet that provides sufficient calories, protein, and carbohydrates to fuel training and recovery.
Hydration: Stay well-hydrated by drinking plenty of fluids throughout the day.
Sleep: Aim for 7-9 hours of quality sleep each night.
Stress Management: Engage in activities such as yoga, meditation, or spending time in nature to reduce stress levels.

Recognizing the signs of overtraining is essential for athletes and fitness enthusiasts to maintain optimal health and performance. By understanding the symptoms, implementing prevention strategies, and addressing overtraining promptly, individuals can avoid potential health risks and achieve their fitness goals safely and effectively.

Chapter 12: Addressing Common Upper Body Concerns

12.1 Targeting Specific Issues: Neck Pain, Rounded Shoulders, etc.

The human body is a complex and interconnected system, and when one part is out of alignment or functioning improperly, it can have ripple effects throughout the body. Two common musculoskeletal issues that many people experience are neck pain and rounded shoulders. While these conditions can be caused by a variety of factors, they often share similar underlying causes and can be effectively addressed through targeted exercises and lifestyle modifications.

Neck Pain

Neck pain is an extremely common condition, affecting up to 70% of adults at some point in their lives. The pain can range from a dull ache to a sharp, stabbing sensation and can be localized to a specific area or radiate down the shoulders and arms. Neck pain can be caused by a variety of factors, including:

Poor posture: 長時間保持不良姿勢，例如駝背或頭部前傾，會給頸部肌肉帶來額外的壓力，導致疼痛和僵硬。
Muscle strain or injury:
頸部肌肉過度使用或受傷也會導致疼痛。這可能是由於不良的睡眠姿勢、重複的動作或創傷造成的。
Degenerative changes:
隨著年齡的增長，頸椎間的椎間盤會開始退化，這會導致疼痛和僵硬。
Underlying medical conditions:
某些潛在的醫療狀況，例如關節炎或纖維肌痛，也會導致頸部疼痛。

Rounded Shoulders

Rounded shoulders, also known as kyphosis, is a condition in which the shoulders are hunched forward and the upper back is rounded. This can give the appearance of a humpback and can lead to pain, stiffness, and decreased range of motion. Rounded shoulders can be caused by a variety of factors, including:

Poor posture: 長時間保持不良姿勢，例如駝背或頭部前傾，會導致頸部和肩部肌肉失去平衡，導致圓肩。
Weak muscles:
頸部和肩部的肌肉力量不足會使它們無法支撐脊柱，從而導致圓肩。
Tight muscles:
胸部和肩部的肌肉過緊會將肩膀向前拉，導致圓肩。
Structural abnormalities:
某些結構異常，例如脊柱側彎或脊椎分離，也會導致圓肩。

Targeted Exercises and Lifestyle Modifications

Both neck pain and rounded shoulders can be effectively addressed through targeted exercises and lifestyle modifications. These interventions aim to improve posture, strengthen muscles, and increase flexibility. Some specific exercises that can be beneficial include:

Neck Pain Exercises:

Chin tucks: This exercise helps to strengthen the muscles that support the neck and improve posture. To perform a chin tuck, stand or sit up straight with your shoulders relaxed. Gently tuck your chin towards your chest, hold for a few seconds, and then release. Repeat 10-15 times.
Neck rotations: Neck rotations help to improve range of motion and reduce stiffness. To perform a neck rotation, sit or stand up straight with your shoulders relaxed. Slowly rotate your head to the right, hold for a few seconds, and then rotate to the left. Repeat 10-15 times in each direction.
Shoulder rolls: Shoulder rolls help to improve flexibility and range of motion in the shoulders. To perform a shoulder roll, stand or sit up straight with your arms at your sides. Roll your shoulders forward in a circular motion for 10-15 repetitions, and then reverse direction and roll your shoulders backward for 10-15 repetitions.

Rounded Shoulders Exercises:

Wall slides: This exercise helps to improve posture and strengthen the muscles that support the shoulders. To perform a wall slide, stand facing a wall with your feet hip-width apart. Place your hands on the wall at shoulder height, with your fingers pointing forward. Slowly slide your body down the wall until your chest touches the wall. Hold for a few seconds and then push back up to the starting position. Repeat 10-15 times.
Shoulder squeezes: This exercise helps to strengthen the muscles that support the shoulders. To perform a shoulder squeeze, sit or stand up straight with your shoulders relaxed. Squeeze your shoulder blades together and hold for a few seconds, and then release. Repeat 10-15 times.
Reverse fly: This exercise helps to strengthen the muscles that support the shoulders and improve posture. To

perform a reverse fly, lie facedown on a bench with your feet flat on the floor. Hold dumbbells in each hand and extend your arms out to the sides, with your palms facing each other. Slowly lift your arms up towards your body, squeezing your shoulder blades together at the top of the movement. Lower back down to the starting position and repeat 10-15 times.

In addition to these exercises, there are a number of lifestyle modifications that can help to improve neck pain and rounded shoulders, such as:

Maintaining good posture: It is important to maintain good posture throughout the day, both when sitting and standing. This means keeping your head up, your shoulders back, and your spine straight.
Using ergonomic equipment: Using ergonomic equipment, such as a supportive chair and a desk that is the right height, can help to reduce strain on the neck and shoulders.
Taking breaks: If you spend a lot of time sitting or standing, it is important to take regular breaks to move around and stretch.
Getting regular exercise: Regular exercise can help to strengthen the muscles that support the neck and shoulders and improve flexibility.
Managing stress: Stress can contribute to neck pain and rounded shoulders, so it is important to find healthy ways to manage stress, such as exercise, yoga, or meditation.

By following these tips, you can help to improve your neck pain and rounded shoulders and enjoy a healthier, more comfortable life.

12.2 Tailoring Wall Workouts for Individual Needs

Wall workouts offer a versatile and effective way to enhance fitness and strength, catering to a wide range of individuals with diverse needs and goals. Tailoring wall workouts to specific requirements ensures optimal results and minimizes the risk of injury. This comprehensive guide will explore the key considerations for customizing wall workouts, empowering individuals to design personalized programs that align with their unique aspirations and limitations.

Assessing Individual Needs

A thorough assessment of individual needs is paramount in tailoring wall workouts. This involves considering various factors that may influence workout design and progression:

Fitness Level: Beginners require workouts that emphasize proper technique and gradual progression to avoid strain or injury. Experienced individuals can incorporate more challenging exercises with increased intensity and complexity.

Strength Goals: The choice of exercises and their modifications should reflect the specific strength goals of the individual. For instance, those aiming to build upper body strength may focus on push-up variations, while those seeking core strength may emphasize plank variations.

Mobility Limitations: Individuals with mobility limitations may need modifications to accommodate their range of motion. For example, wall sit exercises can be performed with the feet elevated on a platform to reduce knee flexion and strain.

Injuries and Conditions: Individuals with injuries or

chronic conditions may require specific modifications to avoid exacerbating existing issues. Consulting with a healthcare professional or certified fitness instructor is recommended to determine appropriate exercise adaptations.

Tailoring Workouts

With individual needs assessed, the following strategies can be employed to tailor wall workouts effectively:

Exercise Selection: Choose exercises that target specific muscle groups and align with fitness goals. Consider the individual's strength, mobility, and any limitations.

Exercise Modifications: Modify exercises to make them easier or more challenging as needed. For instance, beginners can start with half-push-ups on a wall, while advanced individuals can progress to full push-ups with added resistance.

Set and Repetition Adjustments: Adjust the number of sets and repetitions to suit the individual's fitness level and strength goals. Beginners may start with 2-3 sets of 10-12 repetitions, while experienced individuals may perform 4-5 sets of 15-20 repetitions or more.

Rest Periods: The duration of rest periods between sets should be tailored to the individual's recovery capacity. Beginners may need longer rest periods (1-2 minutes), while experienced individuals can opt for shorter rest periods (30-60 seconds) for greater intensity.

Progression Plan: Establish a clear progression plan to gradually increase the challenge as the individual gains strength. This may involve adding sets, repetitions, or modifying exercises to more advanced variations.

Monitoring and Adjustment

Regular monitoring and adjustment are crucial to ensure optimal results and minimize the risk of overtraining or injury:

Body Feedback: Pay attention to how the body responds to workouts. Adjust the intensity or duration if excessive soreness, fatigue, or pain is experienced.

Form Check: Maintain proper form throughout the workouts. Seek guidance from a fitness professional if any technique deviations are observed.

Progress Tracking: Track progress by monitoring strength gains, endurance, or flexibility improvements. This data can guide further adjustments to the workout plan.

Additional Considerations

Warm-up and Cool-down: Warm up before each workout and cool down afterward to prepare the body for exercise and promote recovery.

Hydration: Stay well-hydrated by drinking plenty of water before, during, and after workouts.

Listen to the Body: Respect the body's limits and rest when necessary. Avoid pushing through pain or discomfort.

Enjoy the Process: Wall workouts should be enjoyable and motivating. Choose exercises that are engaging and align with personal preferences.

Tailoring wall workouts to individual needs is essential for maximizing fitness outcomes while minimizing the risk of injury. By considering the factors discussed above and following the recommended strategies, individuals can design personalized programs that meet their unique requirements and help them achieve their fitness goals effectively. Remember, consistency, proper form, and listening to the body are key to successful and enjoyable wall workouts.

12.3 Consulting with a Professional for Personalized Guidance

When embarking on the journey of personal growth and self-improvement, it is often invaluable to seek the guidance of a professional. A therapist, counselor, or coach can provide an objective perspective, offer support and encouragement, and help you develop personalized strategies for achieving your goals.

Benefits of Consulting a Professional

Consulting with a professional offers numerous benefits, including:

Personalized guidance: A therapist or coach can tailor their approach to meet your specific needs, goals, and personality. They can help you identify the root causes of your challenges and develop strategies that resonate with your unique circumstances.
Objectivity: Unlike friends or family members, professionals are trained to provide unbiased and non-judgmental support. They can offer a fresh perspective and help you see situations from a different angle.
Accountability: Working with a professional holds you accountable for your progress. They can provide regular check-ins, set goals, and offer encouragement to keep you motivated.

Emotional support: Therapy or coaching sessions provide a safe and confidential space to express your thoughts and feelings. Your therapist or coach can offer empathy and understanding, helping you navigate challenging emotions.
Improved well-being: Consulting with a professional can lead to significant improvements in your overall well-being. Therapy or coaching can help reduce stress, anxiety, and depression, boost self-esteem, and enhance relationships.

Types of Professionals

There are various types of professionals who offer personalized guidance, including:

Therapists: Therapists specialize in treating mental health conditions such as depression, anxiety, and trauma. They use various therapeutic techniques, such as cognitive-behavioral therapy (CBT) and mindfulness, to help clients improve their mental health.
Counselors: Counselors provide support and guidance for individuals and families facing challenges such as divorce, grief, and career changes. They help clients identify and develop coping mechanisms and strategies for navigating difficult situations.
Coaches: Coaches focus on helping individuals achieve specific goals, such as career advancement, personal growth, or relationship improvement. They provide support, accountability, and guidance to help clients stay motivated and make progress towards their objectives.

Finding the Right Professional

Finding the right professional is crucial for a successful therapeutic or coaching relationship. Here are some tips for finding a qualified professional:

Ask for referrals: Get recommendations from trusted sources such as your doctor, friends, or family members.
Research different professionals: Explore the credentials, experience, and specialties of potential professionals. Read online reviews and testimonials.
Schedule consultations: Meet with a few different professionals before making a decision. This allows you to assess their communication style, approach, and whether you feel a connection.
Trust your instincts: Choose a professional who you feel comfortable with and who you believe can effectively support you on your journey.

Getting the Most Out of Therapy or Coaching

To maximize the benefits of consulting with a professional, it is important to:

Be open and honest: Share your thoughts, feelings, and goals openly with your therapist or coach. The more information they have, the better they can tailor their guidance to your needs.
Be committed: Attend your sessions regularly and actively participate in the process. The more effort you put in, the more likely you are to achieve your desired outcomes.
Follow through: Implement the strategies and recommendations provided by your therapist or coach outside of your sessions. Practice what you learn to see tangible progress in your life.
Be patient: Change takes time. Don't expect to see results overnight. Be patient with yourself and the process, and trust that you will make progress gradually.

Consulting with a professional for personalized guidance can be a transformative experience. By working with a qualified therapist, counselor, or coach, you can gain valuable insights, develop effective strategies, and achieve lasting improvements in your well-being and personal growth.

Chapter 13: Maximizing Your Results

13.1 Building a Mind-Body Connection

The human experience is a symphony of interconnected elements, where the mind, body, and spirit intertwine to create a holistic tapestry of being. The mind, with its cognitive abilities, emotions, and beliefs, exerts a profound influence on the physical realm, while the body, with its intricate physiological systems, provides a tangible expression of our mental and emotional states. Understanding and cultivating the mind-body connection is paramount to achieving optimal well-being and unlocking our full potential.

Unveiling the Mind-Body Axis

The mind-body connection manifests itself in a myriad of ways. Our thoughts and emotions can trigger physiological responses, such as increased heart rate, muscle tension, and hormonal fluctuations. Conversely, physical sensations and bodily experiences can shape our mental and emotional states. For example, pain can lead to anxiety and depression, while exercise can enhance mood and cognitive function. This bidirectional relationship underscores the profound interdependence of the mind and body.

The Science of Mind-Body Integration

Numerous scientific studies have illuminated the intricate

mechanisms underlying the mind-body connection. For instance, research in the field of psychoneuroimmunology has revealed that psychological stress can suppress immune function, increasing susceptibility to infections. Conversely, mindfulness meditation has been shown to strengthen the immune system, promoting health and resilience.

Neuroimaging techniques have also provided valuable insights into the neural pathways involved in mind-body interactions. When we experience physical sensations, specific brain regions involved in sensory processing are activated. However, when we consciously attend to these sensations, additional brain areas associated with emotion, cognition, and self-awareness become engaged, indicating the multifaceted nature of mind-body integration.

Nurturing the Mind-Body Connection

Cultivating a robust mind-body connection is an ongoing practice that requires conscious effort and commitment. Here are some evidence-based strategies to foster this integration:

Mindfulness Meditation: Practicing mindfulness involves paying attention to the present moment without judgment. By cultivating awareness of bodily sensations, thoughts, and emotions, mindfulness strengthens the mind-body connection and promotes emotional regulation, cognitive flexibility, and stress reduction.

Yoga and Tai Chi: These ancient mind-body practices combine physical postures, breathing exercises, and meditation. They enhance flexibility, balance, and cardiovascular health, while also promoting mental calmness, focus, and emotional well-being.

Massage Therapy: Massage can alleviate muscle tension, reduce pain, and improve circulation. It also stimulates the release of endorphins, which have mood-boosting and stress-reducing effects.

Adequate Sleep: Sufficient sleep is essential for both physical and mental recovery. When we sleep, our bodies repair tissues, consolidate memories, and regulate hormone levels. Sleep deprivation can impair cognitive function, increase inflammation, and disrupt the mind-body connection.

Healthy Nutrition: Nourishing our bodies with a balanced diet provides the building blocks for optimal physical and mental health. Consuming whole, unprocessed foods rich in fruits, vegetables, whole grains, and lean proteins supports both our physical and mental well-being.

Benefits of a Strengthened Mind-Body Connection

Integrating the mind and body offers a plethora of benefits for our physical, mental, and emotional health. Some of the well-documented advantages include:

Reduced Stress and Anxiety: Mind-body practices have been shown to effectively reduce stress levels, alleviate anxiety, and promote emotional resilience.

Improved Mood: Engaging in mind-body activities can enhance mood, reduce symptoms of depression, and foster a sense of well-being.

Pain Management: Mind-body techniques can help manage chronic pain by reducing inflammation, improving mobility, and providing coping mechanisms.

Enhanced Cognitive Function: Mindfulness practices have

been linked to improved attention, memory, and decision-making abilities.

Increased Self-Awareness: Mind-body integration promotes self-awareness by fostering a deeper understanding of our thoughts, emotions, and bodily sensations.

Conclusion

Building a robust mind-body connection is an investment in our holistic well-being. By embracing evidence-based practices that nurture this integration, we can unlock the transformative power of the mind and body to achieve optimal health, happiness, and fulfillment. May we all embark on this journey with curiosity, commitment, and a deep appreciation for the interconnected nature of our being.

13.2 Setting Realistic Goals and Tracking Progress

Establishing attainable goals and diligently tracking progress are integral components of achieving any endeavor's desired outcomes. This process enables individuals to maintain focus, stay motivated, and make necessary adjustments along the way. However, the key to success lies in setting realistic goals that align with one's capabilities and resources.

The Importance of Realistic Goals

Unrealistic goals can be detrimental to progress. They often lead to frustration, discouragement, and ultimately, abandonment of the pursuit. By setting realistic goals, individuals can avoid these pitfalls and establish a foundation for sustainable success. Realistic goals are achievable with the effort and resources at one's disposal, and they provide a sense of accomplishment as they are met.

Steps to Set Realistic Goals

Setting realistic goals involves a systematic approach that considers both internal and external factors.

1. Self-Assessment: Begin by evaluating your strengths, weaknesses, skills, and resources. Identify areas where you excel and those that may require further development.
2. Research and Exploration: Gather information about the desired outcome. Consult with experts, read books, or attend workshops to gain insights and identify potential obstacles.
3. Break Down Goals: Divide large, complex goals into smaller, manageable steps. This makes them seem less daunting and allows for gradual progress.
4. Set Timelines: Establish realistic deadlines for each step and the overall goal. Avoid setting overly ambitious timelines that may lead to stress and burnout.
5. Flexibility: Recognize that circumstances may change, and be prepared to adjust goals and timelines accordingly.

Tracking Progress: A Path to Success

Tracking progress is essential for staying on track and making necessary adjustments. Regular monitoring allows individuals to identify areas where they are excelling and areas that require improvement. This information can then be used to refine goals, strategies, and tactics.

Methods for Tracking Progress

Various methods can be employed to track progress

effectively.

1. Journals and Planners: Regularly record your progress, including milestones reached, challenges encountered, and lessons learned.
2. Spreadsheets and Data Tracking Tools: Utilize technology to create spreadsheets or use online tools to track specific metrics and data points related to your goals.
3. Progress Reports: Create periodic reports that summarize your achievements, identify areas for improvement, and outline plans for the next steps.
4. Feedback from Others: Seek feedback from mentors, colleagues, or peers to gain external perspectives and identify blind spots.

Benefits of Tracking Progress

Tracking progress offers numerous benefits, including:

1. Accountability: Regular monitoring holds you accountable for your actions and helps you stay focused on your goals.
2. Motivation: Seeing tangible evidence of progress can boost motivation and keep you inspired to continue striving for success.
3. Course Correction: Tracking progress allows you to identify areas where adjustments are necessary, ensuring that you remain on the path to achieving your goals.
4. Celebration of Successes: Acknowledge and celebrate milestones reached along the way. This helps build confidence and reinforces the value of your efforts.

Conclusion

Setting realistic goals and tracking progress are indispensable tools for achieving success. By following the steps outlined in this one, you can establish goals that align with your capabilities and resources, and you can develop a system for monitoring your progress effectively. Embrace this process to stay motivated, make necessary adjustments, and ultimately reach your desired outcomes.

13.3 Staying Motivated and Committed

Staying motivated and committed is essential for achieving any goal, whether it's completing a task, pursuing a passion, or making a significant life change. However, staying motivated can be challenging, especially when faced with setbacks, distractions, or a lack of support. In this one, we will explore effective strategies for maintaining motivation and staying committed to your goals.

Understanding Motivation

Motivation is the driving force behind our actions. It's what compels us to pursue our goals and overcome obstacles. There are two main types of motivation: intrinsic motivation, which comes from within, and extrinsic motivation, which comes from external factors.

Intrinsic motivation is derived from personal enjoyment, interest, or a sense of accomplishment. When you're intrinsically motivated, you engage in activities because you find them inherently rewarding. This type of motivation is often sustainable and can lead to greater satisfaction and fulfillment.

Extrinsic motivation is influenced by external rewards or punishments. When you're extrinsically motivated, you engage in activities to obtain rewards or avoid consequences. This type of motivation can be effective for short-term goals, but it can be less sustainable and may lead to burnout in the long run.

Strategies for Staying Motivated

1. Set Realistic Goals: Setting achievable goals is crucial for staying motivated. Avoid setting goals that are too ambitious or overwhelming, as this can lead to discouragement and setbacks. Break down large goals into smaller, manageable steps, making them seem less daunting.

2. Identify Your "Why": Determine why your goals are important to you. This could be personal fulfillment, achieving a specific outcome, or making a positive impact on others. Having a clear understanding of your "why" will provide you with intrinsic motivation and help you stay on track even when faced with challenges.

3. Create a Support System: Surround yourself with people who believe in you and support your goals. Share your aspirations with trusted friends, family members, or a mentor. Their encouragement and support can provide you with a sense of accountability and boost your motivation.

4. Visualize Success: Spend time visualizing yourself achieving your goals. Imagine the positive outcomes and the feeling of accomplishment. This can help you stay focused and motivated, even when faced with setbacks.

5. Celebrate Successes: Acknowledge and celebrate your accomplishments along the way. No matter how small, take the time to recognize your progress. This will boost your confidence and keep you motivated to continue working towards your goals.

6. Learn from Setbacks: Setbacks are inevitable. When you

encounter them, don't give up. Instead, learn from your mistakes and adjust your approach. Setbacks can provide valuable insights and help you develop resilience.

7. Stay Positive: A positive mindset is essential for staying motivated. Focus on the progress you're making, no matter how small. Avoid dwelling on setbacks or negative thoughts. Surround yourself with positive people and activities that uplift your spirits.

8. Reward Yourself: When you accomplish significant milestones, reward yourself with something you enjoy. This could be a small treat, a relaxing activity, or spending time with loved ones. Rewarding yourself can provide positive reinforcement and keep you motivated.

9. Take Breaks: Regular breaks are important for maintaining focus and motivation. Step away from your work or activities and engage in something enjoyable and relaxing. This will help you recharge and return to your goals with renewed energy.

10. Practice Self-Discipline: Developing self-discipline is crucial for staying committed to your goals. Establish a routine, set priorities, and stick to your schedule as much as possible. Self-discipline will help you overcome distractions and stay on track, even when you don't feel motivated.

Remember, staying motivated and committed is an ongoing process. There will be times when your motivation wanes. However, by implementing these strategies, you can cultivate a mindset that will help you stay focused, overcome challenges, and achieve your goals.

Chapter 14: Beyond the Wall: Exploring Other Pilates Exercises

14.1 Introducing Mat Pilates for Enhanced Upper Body Strength

Introduction

Pilates, a mind-body exercise method developed by Joseph Pilates in the early 20th century, has gained widespread popularity due to its effectiveness in improving core strength, flexibility, and posture. While traditional Pilates exercises primarily target the core and lower body, variations such as mat Pilates incorporate movements that specifically enhance upper body strength. This one delves into the principles and benefits of mat Pilates for developing a stronger upper body.

Understanding Mat Pilates

Mat Pilates is a form of Pilates that is performed on a cushioned mat, without the use of specialized equipment. The exercises emphasize controlled movements, precise breathing, and maintaining proper alignment throughout the body. Mat Pilates exercises engage various muscle groups, including those in the upper body, core, and lower body.

Benefits of Mat Pilates for Upper Body Strength

Regular practice of mat Pilates offers numerous benefits for enhancing upper body strength, including:

Improved Shoulder Stability: Mat Pilates exercises challenge the shoulder muscles to maintain stability and control during movements. This helps strengthen the muscles around the shoulder joint, reducing the risk of injuries and improving overall shoulder function.
Increased Arm Strength: Many mat Pilates exercises involve pushing, pulling, and lifting motions, which effectively target the muscles in the arms. These movements help develop strength in the biceps, triceps, and forearms, contributing to improved upper body power and endurance.
Enhanced Core Strength: The core muscles play a crucial role in supporting and stabilizing the upper body during movements. Mat Pilates exercises engage the abdominal and back muscles, strengthening the core and providing a solid foundation for upper body exercises.
Improved Posture: Mat Pilates emphasizes maintaining proper alignment throughout the body, which helps correct postural imbalances and reduce muscle imbalances. Improved posture can enhance upper body strength by allowing the muscles to work more efficiently.
Reduced Risk of Injuries: By strengthening the muscles around the joints, mat Pilates helps reduce the risk of injuries in the upper body, such as rotator cuff tears and shoulder impingements.

Incorporating Mat Pilates for Upper Body Strength

To incorporate mat Pilates into a routine for enhanced upper body strength, follow these guidelines:

Start Gradually: Begin with a few basic mat Pilates exercises and gradually increase the intensity and complexity as you become stronger.

Focus on Technique: Prioritize proper form over speed or repetitions. Ensure that your movements are controlled and aligned to maximize the benefits and minimize the risk of injuries.

Engage Your Core: Remember to engage your core muscles during upper body exercises to provide stability and support.

Breathe Deeply: Breathing is an integral part of Pilates. Inhale deeply as you prepare for movements and exhale as you exert effort.

Listen to Your Body: Rest when needed and avoid pushing yourself too hard. If you experience any pain or discomfort, consult with a qualified Pilates instructor.

Conclusion

Mat Pilates is an effective and versatile exercise method that offers numerous benefits for enhancing upper body strength. By incorporating mat Pilates exercises into a regular fitness routine, individuals can improve shoulder stability, increase arm strength, strengthen their core, correct posture, and reduce the risk of injuries. With proper technique, guidance from qualified instructors, and consistency in practice, mat Pilates can help individuals achieve a stronger and more balanced upper body.

14.2 Exploring Equipment Options: Reformer, Cadillac, etc.

The realm of Pilates equipment extends beyond the ubiquitous mat, offering a diverse range of specialized apparatus that cater to varying needs and fitness goals. Each piece of equipment possesses unique characteristics and functionalities, inviting practitioners to explore the intricacies of movement and delve deeper into the Pilates method.

14.2.1 The Reformer

The Reformer, an iconic Pilates apparatus, stands as a versatile training tool that fosters both strength and flexibility. Its centerpiece is a sliding carriage that moves along a frame, allowing for exercises to be performed in a controlled and assisted manner. The Reformer's adjustable springs provide varying levels of resistance, accommodating a wide range of fitness levels.

With the Reformer, practitioners can engage in exercises that target the core, improve posture, enhance balance, and increase mobility. The carriage's smooth gliding action promotes efficient muscle engagement, while the adjustable springs allow for gradual progression in resistance. Whether used for rehabilitation, injury prevention, or athletic performance enhancement, the Reformer offers a comprehensive workout experience.

14.2.2 The Cadillac

The Cadillac, also known as the Trapeze Table, is a sophisticated apparatus that combines elements of the Reformer with additional features that elevate its functionality. The Cadillac features a sturdy frame with a movable carriage, as well as a variety of bars, handles, and straps.

This versatile equipment enables practitioners to explore a wide range of exercises that challenge balance, coordination, and flexibility. The Cadillac's overhead bars allow for exercises that strengthen the upper body and improve spinal alignment. Its adjustable straps and handles facilitate exercises that target the legs, core, and hips.

The Cadillac's unique design makes it particularly suitable for individuals seeking to improve balance and mobility, as well as those recovering from injuries. Its versatility and adaptability cater to a diverse range of needs, making it a valuable addition to any Pilates studio.

14.2.3 The Wunda Chair

The Wunda Chair, a compact yet powerful piece of Pilates equipment, is designed to challenge core strength, stability, and balance. It consists of a cushioned seat with adjustable pedals and a variety of springs.

The Wunda Chair's unique design allows for exercises that isolate specific muscle groups, including the core, hips, and thighs. The adjustable pedals enable practitioners to customize the resistance level, ensuring a tailored workout experience.

This versatile apparatus is ideal for those seeking to enhance core strength and stability. Its compact size makes it suitable for home use or small studios, offering a convenient and effective way to incorporate Pilates into a fitness routine.

14.2.4 The Spine Corrector

The Spine Corrector, a specialized Pilates apparatus, is designed to promote proper spinal alignment and improve posture. It consists of a padded platform with adjustable bars and straps.

With the Spine Corrector, practitioners can perform exercises that gently stretch and mobilize the spine. The adjustable bars and straps provide support and stability, facilitating exercises that target the muscles surrounding the spine.

The Spine Corrector is particularly beneficial for individuals with back pain or imbalances. Its targeted exercises help to improve posture, reduce tension, and enhance spinal health.

14.2.5 The Ladder Barrel

The Ladder Barrel, a unique and challenging Pilates apparatus, combines elements of the Reformer and Cadillac to create a versatile training tool. It features a barrel-shaped frame with a ladder-like structure and adjustable springs.

The Ladder Barrel offers a wide range of exercises that target the core, improve balance, and enhance flexibility. Its curved shape allows for exercises that gently stretch and mobilize the spine. The adjustable springs provide varying levels of resistance, catering to different fitness levels.

This apparatus is particularly suitable for those seeking to improve their posture and flexibility. Its unique design and functionality make it a valuable addition to any Pilates studio, offering a challenging and effective workout experience.

14.2.6 Choosing the Right Equipment

The selection of Pilates equipment should be guided by individual needs, fitness goals, and experience level. It is recommended to consult with a certified Pilates instructor who can assess your specific requirements and provide guidance on the most appropriate equipment options.

Consider the following factors when selecting Pilates equipment:

Fitness goals: Determine whether you are seeking to improve strength, flexibility, balance, or posture. Different equipment options cater to specific fitness goals.
Experience level: Select equipment that is appropriate for your current fitness level and experience with Pilates. Avoid equipment that is too challenging or too basic.
Physical limitations: If you have any physical limitations or injuries, consult with your doctor or a certified Pilates instructor to determine the most suitable equipment options.
Space availability: Consider the available space in your home or studio when selecting equipment. Some apparatus, such as the Cadillac, require more space than others.

By carefully considering these factors, you can make an informed decision that will enhance your Pilates practice and support your fitness journey.

14.3 Building a Comprehensive Pilates Practice

Pilates is a mind-body exercise system that emphasizes core strength, flexibility, and balance. It was developed by Joseph Pilates in the early 20th century and has since become a popular form of exercise for people of all ages and fitness levels.

A comprehensive Pilates practice includes a variety of exercises that target all of the major muscle groups. These exercises are typically performed on a mat or using specialized equipment, such as the Pilates reformer, Cadillac, and Wunda chair.

The benefits of Pilates are numerous and well-documented. Pilates can help to:

Improve posture and alignment
Strengthen the core muscles
Increase flexibility and range of motion
Reduce pain and stiffness
Improve balance and coordination
Promote relaxation and stress relief

Pilates is a safe and effective form of exercise for most people. However, it is important to start slowly and gradually increase the intensity and duration of your workouts as you get stronger. It is also important to find a qualified Pilates instructor who can teach you the proper form and technique.

If you are new to Pilates, it is important to start with a beginner class. This will help you to learn the basics of Pilates and avoid injury. Once you have mastered the basics, you can progress to more advanced classes.

There are many different Pilates studios and classes available. It is important to find a studio that offers classes that are appropriate for your fitness level and goals. You should also make sure that the studio is clean and well-maintained.

Pilates is a great way to improve your overall health and well-being. If you are looking for a safe, effective, and enjoyable form of exercise, Pilates is a great option.

Here are some tips for building a comprehensive Pilates practice:

Start slowly and gradually increase the intensity and duration of your workouts as you get stronger.
Find a qualified Pilates instructor who can teach you the

proper form and technique.
Start with a beginner class if you are new to Pilates.
Find a studio that offers classes that are appropriate for your fitness level and goals.
Make sure that the studio is clean and well-maintained.
Be patient and consistent with your Pilates practice. It takes time to see results.

Here are some sample Pilates exercises that you can try:

The Hundred: This exercise strengthens the abdominal muscles. Lie on your back with your knees bent and your feet flat on the floor. Lift your head and shoulders off the floor and reach your arms overhead. Begin pumping your arms up and down while keeping your core engaged. Do 100 repetitions.
The Roll-Up: This exercise strengthens the abdominal muscles and the hip flexors. Lie on your back with your knees bent and your feet flat on the floor. Lift your head and shoulders off the floor and reach your arms overhead. Then, slowly roll up your spine, vertebra by vertebra, until you are sitting upright. Lower back down to the starting position and repeat. Do 10-15 repetitions.
The Swan Dive: This exercise strengthens the back muscles and the hamstrings. Lie on your stomach with your arms at your sides. Lift your head and chest off the floor and reach your arms overhead. Then, slowly lower your body down towards the floor, keeping your legs straight. Raise your body back up to the starting position and repeat. Do 10-15 repetitions.
The Side Plank: This exercise strengthens the core muscles and the obliques. Lie on your side with your legs stacked on top of each other. Prop yourself up on your elbow and lift your hips off the floor. Hold the position for 30-60 seconds. Repeat on the other side.
The Bridge: This exercise strengthens the buttocks and the hamstrings. Lie on your back with your knees bent and

your feet flat on the floor. Lift your hips up towards the ceiling, squeezing your buttocks at the top of the movement. Lower back down to the starting position and repeat. Do 10-15 repetitions.

These are just a few examples of Pilates exercises. There are many other exercises that you can try, depending on your fitness level and goals. Talk to your Pilates instructor to learn more about Pilates and to create a workout plan that is right for you.

Chapter 15: Maintaining Strength and Sculpting a Defined Physique

15.1 Incorporating Wall Workouts into a Long-Term Routine

Wall workouts offer a versatile and effective way to enhance strength, flexibility, and balance. By leveraging the wall as a stable and supportive surface, individuals can engage in a wide range of exercises that target various muscle groups and movement patterns. To successfully incorporate wall workouts into a long-term routine, it is crucial to adhere to a structured approach that ensures consistency, progression, and injury prevention.

Building a Foundation

Before embarking on a wall workout regimen, it is essential to establish a solid foundation of fitness. This includes developing a baseline level of strength, flexibility, and body awareness. Beginners should start with simple exercises that focus on proper form and technique. As proficiency increases, the intensity and complexity of the workouts can be gradually elevated. Incorporating warm-up and cool-down exercises is also vital to prepare the body for the demands of the workout and promote recovery.

Establishing a Regular Schedule

Consistency is paramount in any fitness routine, and wall workouts are no exception. Establish a regular schedule for your workouts and stick to it as closely as possible. Initially, aim for two to three sessions per week, gradually increasing the frequency as you progress. Be patient and persistent; the benefits of wall workouts will become more apparent over time.

Progressing Gradually

As you become more comfortable with the basic exercises, it is important to challenge yourself to progress. This can be achieved by increasing the duration of your workouts, adding variations to the exercises, or incorporating more challenging movements. Listen to your body and avoid overexertion; progress should be gradual and sustainable to prevent injury.

Listening to Your Body

Paying attention to your body's signals is crucial in any exercise program. If you experience any pain or discomfort during a wall workout, stop the exercise immediately and consult a healthcare professional. Pushing through pain can lead to injuries that may hinder your progress. Rest and recovery are integral parts of any fitness routine; allow your body adequate time to recuperate between workouts.

Variation and Enjoyment

To maintain motivation and prevent boredom, incorporate variety into your wall workouts. Explore different exercises that target various muscle groups and movement patterns. Make the workouts enjoyable by choosing exercises that you find engaging. If you are not enjoying your workouts, you are less likely to stick with them.

Additional Considerations

Proper Form: Maintaining proper form throughout the exercises is essential for maximizing results and minimizing the risk of injury. If unsure about the correct technique, consult with a qualified fitness professional or refer to reputable online resources.
Hydration: Staying hydrated is crucial during any exercise. Drink plenty of water before, during, and after your wall workouts to maintain optimal performance and prevent dehydration.
Appropriate Footwear: Wear supportive and comfortable footwear that provides stability and traction during wall workouts. Avoid shoes with slippery soles or high heels that may increase the risk of injury.
Warm-Up and Cool-Down: Begin each workout with a 5-10 minute warm-up to prepare your body for the exercises. Similarly, conclude each workout with a cool-down routine that includes stretching to promote flexibility and reduce muscle soreness.
Safety: Always ensure that the wall you are using for your workouts is stable and secure. Avoid working out near sharp objects or in areas with uneven surfaces.

Conclusion

Incorporating wall workouts into a long-term routine can provide numerous benefits for individuals of all fitness levels. By adhering to a structured approach that emphasizes consistency, progression, and injury prevention, you can harness the power of wall workouts to enhance your strength, flexibility, and balance. Remember to listen to your body, incorporate variety, and make the workouts enjoyable to maximize your results and sustain your fitness journey.

15.2 Preventing Muscle Loss and Maintaining Gains

The inexorable march of time brings with it an inevitable decline in muscle mass, a condition known as sarcopenia. This gradual loss of muscle tissue not only compromises physical strength and mobility but also increases the risk of falls, fractures, and other debilitating conditions. However, understanding the mechanisms underlying sarcopenia and implementing targeted interventions can effectively mitigate muscle loss and maintain hard-earned gains.

The Causes of Sarcopenia

Sarcopenia results from an imbalance between muscle protein synthesis and breakdown. As we age, several factors contribute to this imbalance:

Reduced protein synthesis: The body's ability to synthesize new muscle proteins diminishes with age due to a decline in growth hormone production and impaired signaling pathways.
Increased protein breakdown: Age-related changes in hormone levels, such as elevated cortisol and reduced testosterone, promote muscle protein breakdown.
Oxidative stress: Free radicals, unstable molecules that damage cells, accumulate with age and contribute to muscle damage and loss.
Physical inactivity: Sedentary lifestyles accelerate muscle loss by reducing the mechanical stimulus necessary for muscle growth and maintenance.
Nutritional deficiencies: Inadequate protein and calorie intake, common among older adults, can impair muscle protein synthesis.

Preventing Muscle Loss

Preventing sarcopenia involves addressing the underlying causes:

Regular Resistance Exercise: Weightlifting, resistance bands, and other forms of resistance training stimulate muscle protein synthesis and minimize breakdown. Aim for 2-3 sessions per week, focusing on compound exercises that engage multiple muscle groups.
Adequate Protein Intake: Protein is essential for muscle growth and repair. Older adults should aim for a daily protein intake of 1.2-1.6 grams per kilogram of body weight, distributed evenly throughout the day. Choose lean protein sources such as fish, chicken, beans, and tofu.
Nutritional Supplementation: Creatine, a naturally occurring compound, has been shown to enhance muscle strength and size. Beta-hydroxy beta-methylbutyrate (HMB), a metabolite of the amino acid leucine, may also support muscle protein synthesis.
Managing Oxidative Stress: Antioxidants, such as vitamin C, vitamin E, and CoQ10, can neutralize free radicals and protect muscle tissue from damage.
Maintaining Physical Activity: Engaging in regular physical activity, including aerobic exercise, helps maintain muscle mass and improves overall health. Aim for at least 150 minutes of moderate-intensity exercise or 75 minutes of vigorous-intensity exercise per week.
Hormone Replacement Therapy: In some cases, hormone replacement therapy with growth hormone or testosterone may be considered to mitigate age-related muscle loss.

Maintaining Muscle Gains

Once you have achieved your desired muscle mass, maintaining it requires ongoing effort:

Consistency with Resistance Exercise: Continue with your

resistance training regimen to stimulate muscle protein synthesis and prevent muscle loss. Gradually increase the weight or resistance as needed to challenge your muscles.
Continued Adequate Protein Intake: Maintain a high protein intake to support muscle repair and growth. Consider adding protein shakes or bars to your diet if meeting your daily protein needs through food alone is challenging.
Progressive Overload: Gradually increase the intensity or duration of your workouts over time to continue challenging your muscles and promoting growth.
Recovery and Rest: Allow for adequate rest and recovery between workouts to facilitate muscle repair and growth. Aim for 7-9 hours of sleep per night.
Lifestyle Factors: Maintain a healthy lifestyle, including a balanced diet, regular exercise, and adequate sleep. Manage stress levels through relaxation techniques such as yoga or meditation.

Conclusion

Preventing muscle loss and maintaining muscle gains requires a comprehensive approach that addresses the underlying causes of sarcopenia. By incorporating regular resistance exercise, consuming adequate protein, managing oxidative stress, and maintaining an active lifestyle, you can effectively preserve muscle mass and enjoy a stronger, healthier life as you age. Remember, consistency and a positive mindset are key to achieving and maintaining your fitness goals.

15.3 The Benefits of Continued Pilates Practice

Pilates, a renowned mind-body exercise discipline, offers a transformative approach to achieving optimal physical and mental well-being. Embarking on a journey of continued Pilates practice transcends mere fitness pursuits; it fosters a profound transformation that extends far beyond the confines of the Pilates studio. With consistent dedication, individuals unlock a myriad of long-lasting benefits that enrich their lives in countless ways.

Enhanced Physical Capabilities

Continued Pilates practice empowers individuals with a heightened level of physical prowess. The methodical exercises and controlled movements strengthen and lengthen muscles, improving overall posture, balance, and coordination. By targeting specific muscle groups, Pilates helps sculpt a lean and toned physique, fostering an enhanced sense of body awareness and control. Additionally, the emphasis on flexibility and range of motion promotes joint mobility, reducing the risk of injuries and enhancing athletic performance.

Improved Core Strength and Stability

The Pilates method places paramount importance on developing a strong and stable core, the foundation of the body. Through repetitive exercises that engage the abdominal and back muscles, Pilates strengthens the core, improving posture and reducing the risk of lower back pain. A robust core enhances overall stability, facilitating effortless movement and improved balance, both in daily activities and during demanding physical endeavors.

Increased Flexibility and Range of Motion

Pilates exercises are designed to gradually increase flexibility and range of motion. By systematically stretching and mobilizing joints and muscles, Pilates helps release tension, improve circulation, and enhance overall mobility. This newfound flexibility fosters a greater sense of ease and freedom in everyday movements, reducing the likelihood of strains and injuries.

Reduced Stress and Improved Mental Well-being

Beyond its physical benefits, Pilates practice profoundly impacts mental health. The controlled and rhythmic movements promote relaxation and stress reduction. Pilates encourages individuals to focus on their breathing and body awareness, creating a sense of mindfulness and tranquility. Regular practice has been shown to reduce anxiety levels, improve mood, and enhance overall well-being.

Injury Prevention and Rehabilitation

Pilates is an invaluable tool for injury prevention and rehabilitation. By strengthening core muscles, improving posture, and enhancing flexibility, Pilates reduces the risk of developing common injuries. Additionally, the controlled movements and focus on proper form can aid in the rehabilitation process after an injury, accelerating recovery and preventing re-injury.

Long-term Benefits: A Lifetime of Enhanced Well-being

The benefits of continued Pilates practice extend far into the future, providing individuals with a lifetime of enhanced well-being. By maintaining a consistent Pilates routine, individuals can preserve and even improve their physical and mental capabilities as they age. The strong foundation established through Pilates supports healthy aging, reducing the risk of chronic diseases, falls, and age-related ailments.

Conclusion

Embracing a journey of continued Pilates practice is an investment in oneself, promising a lifetime of physical and mental well-being. The transformative benefits of Pilates extend far beyond the confines of the studio, empowering individuals with a stronger, more flexible, and balanced body, a reduced risk of injuries, and a profound sense of calm and well-being. By consistently dedicating themselves to this transformative discipline, individuals embark on a path towards a healthier, more fulfilling, and vibrant life.

Chapter 16: Conclusion

16.1 Achieving Your Upper Body Strength Goals

Introduction

Developing upper body strength is crucial for numerous activities of daily living, sports performance, and overall well-being. Whether you aim to improve your posture, enhance athletic capabilities, or simply maintain a healthy lifestyle, achieving your upper body strength goals requires a comprehensive approach that encompasses proper training, nutrition, and recovery.

Exercise Selection

The foundation of any strength training program lies in selecting exercises that effectively target the desired muscle groups. For upper body development, a balanced approach should incorporate exercises that work the chest, shoulders, back, and arms. Compound movements, such as bench press, overhead press, and rows, engage multiple muscle groups simultaneously, maximizing efficiency and overall strength gains. Isolation exercises, like bicep curls and tricep extensions, can further refine muscle development and address specific weaknesses.

Progressive Overload

Progressive overload is a fundamental principle of

strength training that involves gradually increasing the resistance or weight lifted over time. As your body adapts to the demands of your workouts, it becomes necessary to provide a greater challenge to continue stimulating muscle growth. This can be achieved by increasing the weight lifted, the number of repetitions performed, or the sets completed. Progressive overload should be implemented consistently and in a controlled manner to avoid plateaus or injuries.

Proper Form and Technique

Maintaining proper form and technique is paramount for maximizing the effectiveness of your workouts and minimizing the risk of injury. Correct form ensures that the targeted muscle groups are being activated efficiently and that excessive stress is not placed on joints and tendons. Pay attention to your posture, body alignment, and the full range of motion for each exercise. If necessary, seek guidance from a qualified fitness professional to refine your technique and ensure optimal results.

Adequate Nutrition

Proper nutrition plays a vital role in supporting your upper body strength training efforts. Consuming a balanced diet that provides adequate protein, carbohydrates, and healthy fats is essential for muscle growth and recovery. Protein is the building block of muscle tissue, and consuming sufficient amounts is crucial for repairing and rebuilding muscles after workouts. Carbohydrates provide the energy needed to fuel your workouts, while healthy fats support hormone production and cell function.

Hydration

Hydration is often overlooked but is equally important for

optimal strength training performance. Water aids in nutrient transport, waste removal, and body temperature regulation. Aim to drink plenty of water throughout the day, especially before, during, and after your workouts. Dehydration can lead to fatigue, decreased muscle function, and an increased risk of injuries.

Recovery

Recovery is an integral component of any strength training program. Allow sufficient time for your body to rest and repair after intense workouts. This includes getting adequate sleep, incorporating rest days into your training schedule, and engaging in active recovery activities, such as light cardio or stretching. Overtraining can hinder progress, increase the risk of injuries, and lead to burnout.

Consistency and Patience

Building upper body strength takes time and consistency. It is important to remain patient and dedicated to your training plan. Results will not appear overnight, but with regular effort and adherence to the principles outlined above, you will gradually achieve your goals. Avoid becoming discouraged by temporary setbacks or plateaus. Instead, view these challenges as opportunities to refine your technique and adjust your training approach.

Additional Tips

- Warm up before each workout with light cardio and dynamic stretching to prepare your body for the exercises ahead.

- Cool down after each workout with static stretching to improve flexibility and reduce muscle soreness.

- Use a spotter when attempting heavy lifts to ensure safety and minimize the risk of injury.

- Listen to your body and take rest days when necessary to prevent overtraining and allow for recovery.

- Consider working with a certified personal trainer for personalized guidance, motivation, and accountability.

Conclusion

Achieving your upper body strength goals requires a comprehensive approach that encompasses proper training, nutrition, and recovery. By incorporating these principles into your routine, you can effectively build strength, improve athletic performance, and enhance your overall well-being. Remember, consistency, patience, and dedication are key to realizing your fitness aspirations.

16.2 Embracing the Power of Pilates for a Stronger, More Defined You

Introduction

In a world where physical fitness and aesthetics often take center stage, the pursuit of a stronger, more defined physique has become a common goal for many individuals. While there are countless ways to achieve this objective, Pilates stands out as a comprehensive and effective approach that can transform not only your body but also your overall well-being.

The Principles of Pilates

Developed by Joseph Pilates in the early 20th century, Pilates is a low-impact, body-conditioning exercise method that focuses on developing core strength, flexibility, balance, and coordination. It emphasizes the importance of proper breathing techniques, precise movements, and maintaining a neutral spine throughout the exercises.

Benefits of Pilates

The benefits of Pilates are numerous and encompass both physical and mental aspects. Regular practice can lead to:

Enhanced core strength, which improves posture, stability, and athletic performance
Increased flexibility, reducing muscle tightness and improving range of motion
Improved balance and coordination, enhancing overall mobility and reducing the risk of falls
Reduced muscle imbalances, leading to better posture and a more defined physique
Improved body awareness and mind-body connection, promoting stress reduction and increased self-confidence

Core Strengthening with Pilates

The core is the powerhouse of the body, and Pilates exercises specifically target this area to develop strength and stability. Core muscles include the abdominals, lower back muscles, and pelvic floor muscles. By engaging these muscles in controlled and precise movements, Pilates strengthens the core and improves overall body function.

Flexibility Enhancement

Pilates exercises incorporate stretching and lengthening movements that increase flexibility throughout the body. This flexibility can reduce muscle tension, improve posture, and enhance athletic performance. It also contributes to a more graceful and fluid movement quality.

Balance and Coordination

Pilates emphasizes balance and coordination through exercises that challenge stability and require precise movements. By maintaining balance and coordinating different body parts, Pilates improves overall body control and reduces the risk of falls.

Muscle Definition

While Pilates is not specifically designed for muscle building, it can effectively define muscles by increasing lean muscle mass and reducing body fat. By focusing on core strength, flexibility, and body awareness, Pilates promotes a balanced and toned physique.

Getting Started with Pilates

To experience the transformative benefits of Pilates, it is recommended to start with a certified Pilates instructor who can guide you through the proper form and techniques. Regular practice is key, with sessions typically lasting between 45 minutes to an hour. Consistency and patience are essential for achieving optimal results.

Conclusion

Embracing the power of Pilates can lead to a stronger, more defined you, both physically and mentally. Through its emphasis on core strength, flexibility, balance, and coordination, Pilates empowers individuals to achieve their fitness goals and enhance their overall well-being. Whether you are a beginner or an experienced athlete, Pilates offers a transformative exercise method that can reshape your body and enrich your life.

16.3 Continuing Your Journey Towards a Fit and Healthy Lifestyle

Sustaining a healthy and active lifestyle is a commendable pursuit that requires ongoing effort and commitment. As you navigate the path towards lifelong well-being, it is essential to recognize that setbacks and challenges may arise. These obstacles should not deter you; rather, they provide opportunities for growth and resilience. Remember that progress is not always linear, and there will be times when you may falter or experience setbacks. The key lies in your unwavering determination to learn from your experiences and continue moving forward, one step at a time.

To maintain a healthy and active lifestyle, it is crucial to establish a structured routine that aligns with your individual needs and preferences. This may involve setting realistic goals, scheduling regular physical activity, and making informed nutritional choices. It is important to find activities that you enjoy and can incorporate into your daily life, whether it's brisk walking, cycling, swimming, or pursuing a hobby that brings you joy. Moreover, mindful eating habits and hydration are essential components of a holistic approach to well-being.

In addition to physical health, mental and emotional well-being play a significant role in your overall health and happiness. Engage in activities that nurture your mental health, such as meditation, yoga, spending time in nature, or pursuing creative outlets. Prioritize sufficient sleep, as it is essential for both physical and cognitive functioning. Moreover, cultivate meaningful relationships with supportive individuals who encourage and inspire you on your health journey.

As you progress on your journey towards a fit and healthy lifestyle, remember that it is a lifelong endeavor that requires consistent effort and adaptation. Regularly assess your progress, make adjustments as needed, and seek professional guidance when necessary. Surround yourself with a supportive network of family, friends, or health professionals who can provide encouragement and accountability. Embrace the process as an ongoing exploration of your body, mind, and spirit, and revel in the benefits of a life lived in pursuit of well-being.

Lastly, always remember that maintaining a fit and healthy lifestyle is not about perfection or unrealistic ideals. It is about making choices that prioritize your overall well-being, honoring your body's needs, and embracing a mindset of self-compassion and acceptance. Celebrate your successes, learn from your setbacks, and approach your health journey with a sense of curiosity, flexibility, and unwavering commitment to living a vibrant and fulfilling life.

Printed in Great Britain
by Amazon